THE COMPANION GUIDE
FOR THE
LOW BACK PAIN PROGRAM

Accelerate The Program To Relieve Your Pain

Learn Additional, Essential, Tips & Techniques

*All The Support You Need To Achieve The Most Success
& Maximize Your Pain Relief*

INCLUDES

**Getting Started: How To Begin When In Pain
*& Are Not Sure What To Do***

Do's & Don'ts Of Relieving Pain While On The Program

ON THE GO: How To Use The Program Anywhere To Relieve Pain

12 Modified Exercises To Help You With The Program

**10 Charts To Relieve Pain At Work, Away, Home,
When Active Or Going To Sleep**

8 Common Back Problems You Can Correct

***15 More Tips & Support* For Protecting Your Back**

**7 Custom *Quick Start Charts* To Tackle Everyday
Concerns That Hurt Your Back**

Over 110 Pages of Support with 100+ Additional Images!

Sherwin A. Nicholson   © 2018   SN Health Resources

The Companion Guide

for The Low Back Pain Program

ISBN 978-1720948797 (eBook)

Contents

Hello & Welcome!

Thank you for using the Companion Guide for The Low Back Pain Program.

To begin, I would like to get you acquainted with what this Guide and the Program are all about. This way, you will be *more prepared* and focused so you can have the most pain relief as possible.

Sometimes, starting the first few exercises *to test out* how well it will help you may seem OK. However, with a little preparation before hand, you can avoid any unnecessary mistakes, be better able to learn the exercises and enjoy them as you begin to feel better.

Also, as I have maintained, I don't want to unnecessarily waste your time as relieving discomfort can be very time sensitive and consuming. So I have only included only what is beneficial for you and *not filler* that you may find irrelevant.

I have listed below the following links to my website for additional support. Whenever you need to contact me, you can reach me at info@lowbackpainprogram.com. I always reply and give support for every email that is sent to me in a timely fashion.

I truly appreciate your interest and use of this Guide and the Program. I am committed to *helping you overcome your pain* as best as I can.

Sincerely,

Sherwin Nicholson, Author.

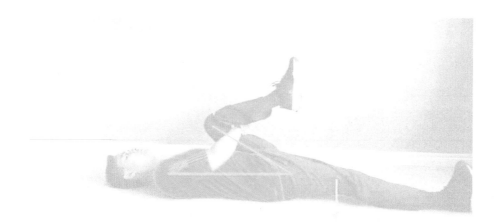

The Low Back Pain Program

Getting You Back On Track

This program *simply put,* is meant to relieve back pain. Specifically, it is meant to recondition you out of the limitations and pain that you have likely developed over many years of possible neglect, strain or injury. If your lifestyle in the past or present has been adding to the discomfort, this guide will help you to make many necessary changes.

Our bodies when younger can naturally bear and tolerate almost any activity we can put it through. It's, not until we have: become progressively over trained from athletics, undertrained from neglect due to work, lack of time or choice, a specific back condition or have been injured, that we develop chronic back issues that can become difficult to overcome.

The good news is that you'll now be learning how to tackle and overcome these specific chronic issues.

One thing that you'll notice is the way I *name* each exercise. *Ex. Seated Leg Opener, Standing Hip Shift...* I avoid using obscure or creative names because I want you to know as easily as possible what you'll be doing. This way, once you get the hang of the exercises, you'll be able to *quickly perform any one* by simply reading from the chart schedules without having to rely on the images.

How the Program Helps You

Each exercise in the program has its own fundamental purpose for making your muscles and joints healthier. Each one serves to release and strengthen a specific area that is very likely causing you pain. *There aren't any exercises in the program that are not helpful.*

Although **45** exercises do seem like a lot, you only need to focus on the ones you'll need *as you go along. This way at any given time, it's only 3 to 4 exercises which you are doing.* You are performing all 45 over a controlled and relaxed period of time instead of all at once (depending on any limitations such as knee pain).

You will be using several techniques to relieve back pain through self-conditioning at *your* pace. There is no pressure to complete all exercises to feel better. *You will feel better much sooner.* However, it does take time and dedication *usually while you are not feeling your best.*

The Low Back Pain Program is a complete program that can be done alone or with support. It comes with numerous tips and free coaching from myself (please email me anytime!) to help you along the way.

The Companion Guide

A Guide to Prepare and Support You

Simply put, this Guide will help you manage and relieve your back pain as effectively as possible *as you manage your daily needs*. It will give you a greater awareness, preparation and focus on how to help take care of your back while being protected.

With this additional support, you can maximize your ability to retrain, recondition and return to the life you want as safely and effectively as possible.

In addition to the exercises and support already in the program, this Guide will help you with specific problems you may have and may come across while on your recovery. You will learn a great deal more about what you can and should be doing *outside* of the daily exercises taught in the program.

You can then learn how to use the exercises in your everyday routines *without wasting time* as you protect your back. It's a *win-win* because you can integrate the program to be part of your life and feel better. *This is more ideal than just practicing it sometimes in the hopes of feeling better.*

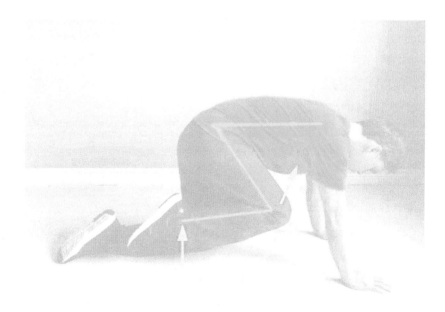

The 3 Challenges of Taking Care of Your Back

Now that you have been able to dedicate your time and energy, *you will need to be prepared for the following concerns.*

When on any new program such as this one, you'll encounter the following:

1) **Your Current Pain.** The chronic muscular or nerve related discomfort that you have now and the limitations *from that pain* that can make you anxious or hesitant. It's normal to be concerned whenever you start something new. If you can reassure yourself that you are on a reconditioning and rehabilitation type program, you'll be more confident.

   Stay focussed on relieving the pain that comes from imbalances and weaknesses that cause muscle, disc and nerve pain. These are temporary and can be healed.

2) **The Discomfort of the New Exercise.** Reconditioning and exercising weak, tight and sore muscles or joints is **not** comfortable. They are not accustomed to the sudden changes and adjustments and are being constantly challenged until they become longer, stronger and more flexible.
   It's this soreness that can alarm people. The reaction may be that they feel more pain but it is likely from the new adjustment you are challenging your body with.

   This is why I only recommend 3-4 exercises at one time at a very slow and gradual pace. It's important to include a rest period to accommodate for these changes.

3) **Pain from a Joint or Disc.** This can include an arthritic joint, ruptured disc or degenerative condition to name at least three. *These painful conditions require the most patience and time to relieve.* The exercises will help to relieve a lot of pain in these areas. However, for fairly advanced conditions, it will be difficult to relieve all of the pain.

   As you develop more strength, flexibility and a greater range of motion, you are using one of the best methods to reduce *the inflammation, swelling and damage* present. The key to relieving this form of pain is by <u>reducing the inflammation</u>.

With these 3 challenges, you may have to cope with just one, two or all of them at once. If you begin to feel overwhelmed on a day where it feels like all three challenges are too much for you, **take a break and rest.** You don't need to be perfect, *only committed.*

Getting the Most Out of the Program and Guide

To get the most effective relief, always remember, *it's about your needs and your body's pace*. It's not a race and there is *no value* in rushing through the Program.

Go through each exercise, slowly and carefully. Because each one can be so different, know that it will help you with a specific limitation that you may have that contributes to your pain. Sometimes you will feel the benefit of the exercise *immediately*, or in many cases, the exercise simply prepares you for the ones *ahead*. So the benefit *does* come.

Difficulty

There will be times where you will find it very hard to do a particular exercise. Don't be alarmed, this is to be expected. Please recognize this *temporary obstacle* as an indication that you have developed a number of imbalances and weakness that restrain you from completing the exercise.

This helps you to evaluate where you must focus your time on to bring back muscle strength, length and flexibility to a specific part of your body. By staying focus and patient, your back is gradually receiving protection and support from the exercise.

Dedication

Much dedication and patience is required. As you know, your back is the priority and that there are no quick fixes. *Your body will recover and heal at its own pace*. This may frustrate you as you wait but remember to remain focused and take your time.

You won't feel as frustrated if you expect sometimes that there may be days where you feel better and days where you are tired or sore. Know that this comes with taking much needed care of yourself while on a good long term program.

Support

Whenever you need help, there is help for you. Not only will the tips and support in the program help, but that is only the beginning. This guide is also here to answer many questions and concerns you may have.

For additional help, you can also go online for the following:

- Frequently Asked Questions of The Program
  https://lowbackpainprogram.com/frequently-asked-questions/
- Commonly Asked Questions from Current Users
  https://lowbackpainprogram.com/ebook-support-faqs/
- eBook/PDF/Program Instructions on How to Use The Program
  https://lowbackpainprogram.com/ebook-instructions/

And most importantly, just send me an email through the contact page anytime. You can also contact me at info@lowbackpainprogram.com. PDF users are given my direct email via my courtesy PDF backup email. I always respond within 1-2 business days and you can email me as much as you need. I am here to help and support you.

Sincerely,

Sherwin Nicholson, Hons.B.Sc.

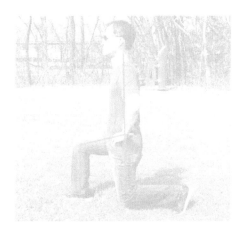

Getting Started:

When You're in Pain and Not Sure What to Do

Beginning what may seem to be such a different and extensive program can be a bit intimidating to say the least.

Let's address some common concerns that you may have.

Compatibility

By now, you may be accustomed to performing very standard exercises and stretches that may or may not have helped you. If your back problems are significant, you are also very likely using the services of a chiropractor, physiotherapist, doctor, etc.

The Program is designed to be used with *any* form of therapy and will not interfere with any other treatments you may be using. The advantage of the program is that it is intended to help you *self train* so that you can take care of your back with or without added treatment.

In most cases you can either continue your current treatment or physical activity along with the Low Back Pain Program or just focus on the Program entirely. Following it alone does allow you to minimize injury or re-injury.

Caveats

Additional support is fine to use when on the Program provided that your *activity is not adding any undo strain to your body*. Some examples would be extreme yoga, martial arts, contact sports or weight training. This would make it more difficult for you to determine whether or not your own activities are a factor in your recovery process.

I don't discourage any activities or sports while on the program. It's OK to stay active. This Program only requires about 10-30 min of practice each day.

Daily Use

Once you really get comfortable with the exercises, you'll find them quite easy to incorporate into your day without taking up much of your time. For example, instead of leaning over, *which is bad for your already sore back,* simply do the Reverse Lunge as taught in the Program. You won't find in very convenient at first but if you commit to it as your new and preferred way to lower yourself, you have not only eliminated a bad habit but have also begun reconditioning and activating your hips and legs.

This keeps you protective and active with less pain. Doing this uses **no** extra time in your day *while at the same time,* you're using the Program!

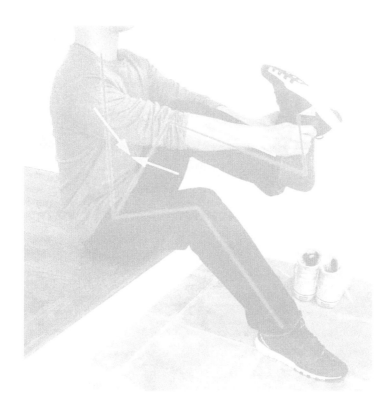

Recommendations on Starting

1) **Stay active**. Don't quit your sports or activities. Most activities are fairly safe for your back in moderation and also help to keep you moving.

2) **Only avoid activities which are not *'back safe'*.** For instance, weight bearing, heavy lifting, excessive bending or twisting movements cause your lumbar curve to go out of neutral curve too often (leaning or arching).

3) **Don't begin if you have a very *sharp* pain sensation**, especially if it radiates down your back or leg. *You must see your doctor and get consent to exercise.* You may have a disc rupture or pinched nerve.

4) **Use padding** such as a pillow or a support wrap if you have knee or hip issues. Some exercises do require effort from these joints. You can either opt out of some of them if you find that they cause strain or continue with them at a later time.

5) **Dress comfortably.** The Program is designed to be done anywhere and anytime. Ideally, a loose fitted pant or shorts are ideal. This allows your hips to open up easier and allows it to move with your lower back. Avoid tight clothing that does not stretch sufficiently for your hips and legs. Your lower body should always be more active than your upper.

The First Exercise: The Deep Squat Rest

This exercise is the first because it will test and reveal your limitations. *The easier that you can move into and out this simple position, the less back pain you will have.*

The goal of squatting deeply is to:

- Bring greater flexibility and range to your hips
- Stretch the calf muscles
- Release tightness in your lower back
- Develop gluteus muscle strength
- Improve your pelvic tilt

Most people never have an opportunity to squat this way. It provides a lot of benefits for your lower back and lower body when you do it often.

It's not easy to squat

Don't worry if at first you have a lot of difficulty performing it. For people with back pain, **this is expected.** It may be hard for you to master but *it is worth it.* Expect for you to take at least a few weeks to finally achieve it.

Your entire lower body and lower back will need to readjust to this position. It always takes a while for anyone's flexibility to improve so patience is vital.

Here are some tips when Deep Squatting:

1) **Hold** on to a support *as you lower* to keep balanced
2) Keep your behind against a **wall** to avoid falling backward
3) Keeping your feet flat on the ground is *not* essential but may indicate very short calf muscles *which also affect your back.*
4) **Stretch** your calf muscles often to help with this squat
5) Lower yourself slowly and **allow gravity** to ease you down
6) Only rely on your legs to raise and lower you
7) You can squat either with your feet apart, close together or both

Knee pain?

If your knees hurt during the Deep Squat Rest, then **you can modify it** by lying on your back and hugging one thigh at a time. Then in time, you can hug both at the same time. **This modification however does not stretch your calves** so be sure *to increase the amount of time* that you dedicate to stretching your calves also.

Don't focus too much on the Deep Squat! *All exercises take time.* The most effective way to benefit is to perform each exercise for **about 1-3 minutes** each at a time and no longer.

How to Schedule Your Exercises

45 exercises may seem like quite a lot but *by breaking them down* into levels and only doing a few at a time, it will become quite easy.

Remember, each exercise is intended to relieve some or a few specific limitations that lead to your pain. This means that you will find a lot of relief well before you complete all of them! *Most programs fail because they just are **not** very convenient to do.* You will now be able to avoid this very common pitfall.

First of all, if you find it very difficult to find time to exercise for about 10 – 20 minutes per day, you're not alone. No one has time. If you do, then *you most likely have had to sacrifice it from somewhere else too!*

Prioritizing

The truth is that too much time is usually spent on fairly low priority tasks (devices). This is where you can take advantage of this available time to get in a minute here and there to follow the Program.

Another way you will be able to schedule you exercises will be by performing them with everyday routines and activities you do now but instead can use the exercise as a substitute.

The **ON THE GO** section of this guide will give you all the higher priority exercises you can do in your regular work and leisure schedule. This will not only <u>save you time</u> but *change the way you keep active* to prevent yourself from suffering any pain that you've developed.

Prioritizing will help you to remain vigilant about your own back health and safety with little effort.

Begin the First 3 Exercises

Start with the first **3** exercises of the **Limited Mobility Program**:

> ### *The Deep Squat Rest, the Kneeling Bow Rest & the Seated Leg Opener.*

They are **all** about *improving your hip mobility and releasing the current tension* in your lower back.

The goal is to loosen up the most tense and stiff areas that are causing you pain. *There is no need to stretch and strengthen anything else at this time.*

It's natural at this time to want instant relief but it can't happen if your body is tight and stiff.

Tight muscles and stiff joints limit your mobility and hurt your back. Any exercises, activities or sports that you engage in when in this vulnerable state *will make things worse for your back.*

The Amount of Time Required

Spend 1 minute per exercise when you begin. Do once in the morning, the afternoon and then finally in the evening.

When you feel comfortable to practice them for a *longer* period of time, extend it to 2 minutes and then 3. It may take several days before you can reach this length of time but that's OK.

By doing 3 different exercises per day for 1 -3 minutes each, every morning, afternoon and evening, you will require 9-27 minutes per day. This is a fairly reasonable amount of time when your back needs treatment.

The times and frequencies that I have recommended are only suggestions of course. *Feel free to modify them to your convenience **as long as you don't overdo it.***

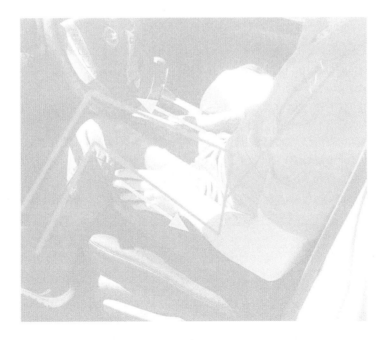

Do's and Don'ts While on the Program

As you practice the exercises, you may have additional concerns that may go beyond the information provided in the eBook/Hardcopy. I have listed below some Do's and Don'ts to help you get the most out of the Program and to avoid any setbacks.

Do:

1) Only **1** level at a time.
2) Up to **3-4** exercises at a time for each level per day (preferably in order).
3) Each exercise up to 3 times per day (morning, afternoon, evening).
4) Spend **1-3 min** per exercise (minimum **9** minutes per day).
5) Each exercise slowly and *only to your range and comfort level.*
6) Use pillows and cushions for padding (ex. Knee support).
7) Add **1** new exercise *when **1** current exercise become fairly easy to do* (you can skip the easy one, perform it much less often or only as needed.
8) Rest often if you feel sore. Each exercise will have a new effect on your flexibility and strength so you may need to take a break to recover. Check out the '3 Challenges'.

Don't:

1) Don't do too many exercises at once. Too many can overstrain your body and back and may set you back. Changes need to be slow and steady. **3** different exercises per day are preferred.
2) Don't force yourself into the final position in the images. You may strain yourself. Just transition slowly day by day.
3) Don't do any exercises if you have a sharp pain. This most likely if from a disc or nerve injury. See your doctor for consent.
4) Skip any exercises where you have specific knee issues. Many exercises will have a caution to protect you. Some back issues such a spondylolisthesis or fusions may limit what you can safely do. In these situations, *your doctor's advice is the priority.*
5) Don't skip any levels. Each levels and exercise helps to prepare you for the next. Skipping may risk injury making your progress less effective.

ON THE GO

How to Use the Program at Work, Away, Home or In Bed

The best way you can feel better is to be able to use many of the exercises anywhere. This is important because you may need relief at any given time. Much of what you do every day can cause pain so there is likely an exercise available to help you.

NOTE: Most of the more advanced exercises outlined below can be done *after you have dedicated enough time* to practicing the easier ones. It is generally better to only use the exercise when you have *progressed to that level.*

What you will be able to do is improve your limited mobility, progress with strengthening & stretching and to then be able to challenge your new flexibility and strength to protect you from harm.

Below are some very typical situations where you may encounter chronic lower back pain and what you can do.

NOTE*: These ON THE GO recommendations are only intended for pain management and should not be done as a substitute for the entire Program.* **It is better to follow the Program and the ON THE GO exercises together to have long term pain relief.**

Listed below are the key exercises you want to do when on the go. You'll find that many activities overlap with one another. There are many listed below to choose from.

If you find that some movements are difficult, this means that your body has developed a muscle and joint imbalance to *limit* that movement. *It is that very limitation that needs to be reconditioned to help your back.*

Note: **For best results, you must first learn the steps of each exercise listed below** *from the Program.* **Only the name and final pose of the exercise is shown below.**

In The Office

Sitting may feel comfortable at first but the more time that you spend in this position, the more your back will suffer. The seated posture causes muscle tightening and weakening. *Your body CANNOT support your back whenever you sit.* Because your office environment severely limits your movement and posture here are some exercises you can still practice.

They will help you to

- activate your leg muscles
- improve blood circulation to the muscles and nerves
- maintain neutral pelvic tilt
- keep your back muscles from weakening
- prevent muscle weakness and tightening

Seated Leg Opener – Keeps your hips open and flexible to provide arch support.

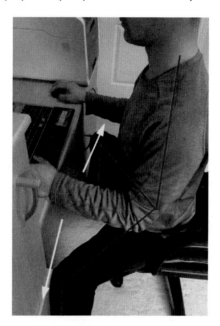

Seated Leg Rotation (assisted with contraction) – Further provides strength and flexibility to release back tension and to activate your glutes.

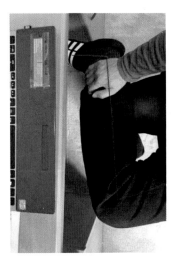 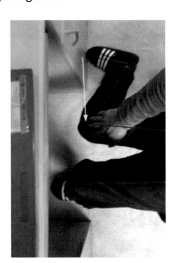

Seated Lunge – A must to keep your hip flexors from becoming tight. Relieves lower back tension and helps keep your back from slouching.

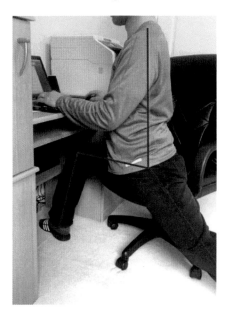

Seated Knee Raise - Keeps your hip flexors active and helps to strengthen your core for back protection.

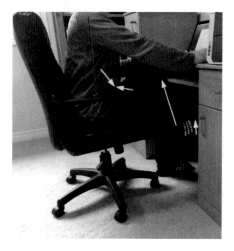

Seated Hip Adjustment – Stops your hips from becoming overly tight and sore. Releases tension in your lower back.

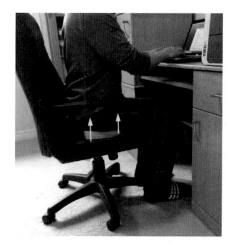

Seated Hip Shift – Keeps your hips active, releases tension and improves your circulation. It stabilizes your core and strengthens very weak hip and back muscle groups. Improves your hip flexibility.

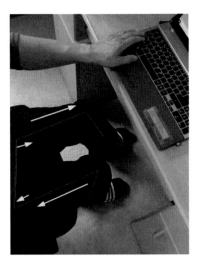

Seated Leg to Chest – Prevents Sciatica and Piriformis pain. Improves gluteus circulation. Relieves lower back tension.

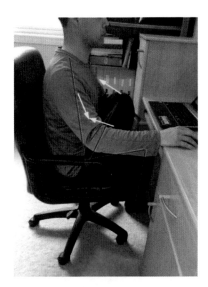

Seated Calf Stretch – Stretches your calf muscles while also strengthening your core. Activates your hip flexors, leg muscles and boosts circulation.

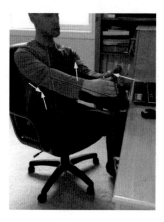

Seated Leg Lifts – Activates and strengthens your legs and core. Improves the circulation in your legs while sitting.

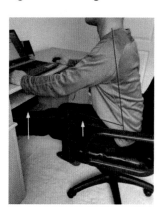 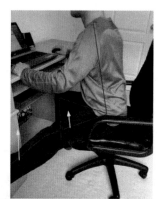 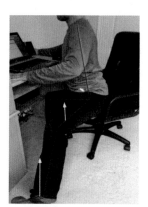

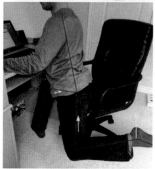

At Home

Around your home, there is a range of exercises that you can take advantage of that can be seamlessly added to your day. *Of course, you don't have to do them well, just often.* In time, you will improve with flexibility and will be able to do them faster.

The following exercises from the program are what you can use depending on the chore or activity you may have.

Deep Squat Rest – A better alternative to other squats. Use whenever you need to be lower to the ground.

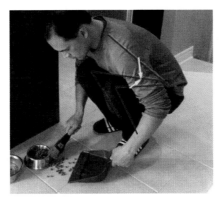

Seated Leg Cross (with or without the forward lean) – Use this seated position when you can lean forward occasionally.

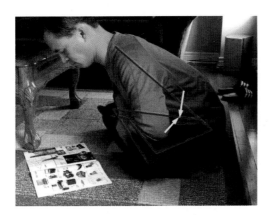 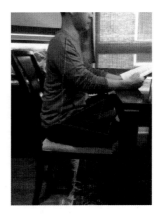

Floor Leg Bend and Shift (also when you are sitting) - When watching TV as a better alternative to sitting on a couch.

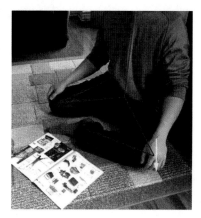 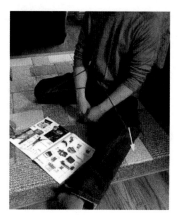

Seated Leg to Chest - Do this anytime you must sit at home to help treat and prevent Piriformis and Sciatic pain.

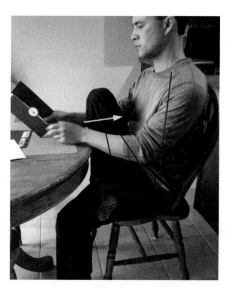

Leaning Hip Shift - Do this at the same time you brush your teeth. It will help to loosen your hips, stretch the hamstrings and activate your leg muscles.

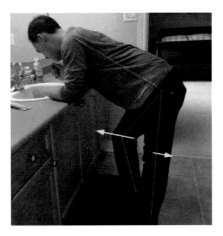

Stair steps – Going upstairs every other step will help you develop your gluteus strength easily. It also saves you time.

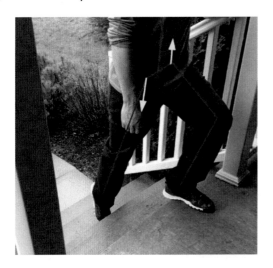 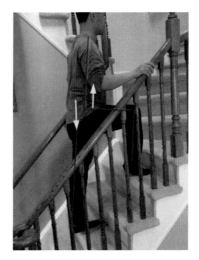

Seated Calf Stretch – This is excellent for when you dress or undress while on the bed or a chair. Example, socks, shoes, underwear, pants etc.

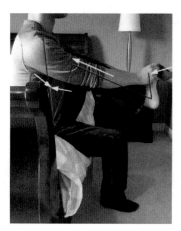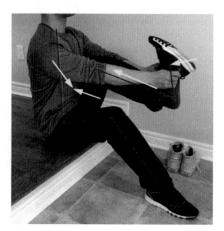

Standing Abdominal – This is an easy movement you can do anytime. It's best to do it when you anticipate having to stand for long periods. It will help you to relieve the lower back tension that standing causes.

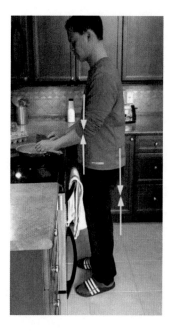

Squat (holds, leans, circles, steps, walks) – This is not always a very convenient exercise to do but it is what conditions your legs and hips to remain both active and supportive. The more you do this exercise, the more stamina you'll have to help relieve your back.

Squat activities at home include: cleaning, vacuuming, shovelling, mowing, carrying items.

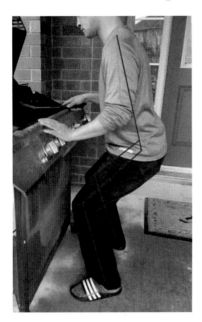
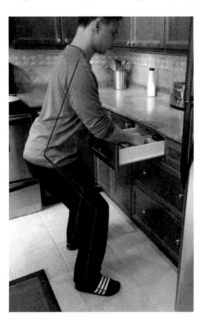

Lunge with Reverse Kneel – Of all of the AT HOME exercises, you'll be doing these the most often. Anytime you need to lower yourself, use it as your preferred method, instead of leaning over.

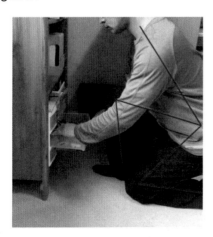
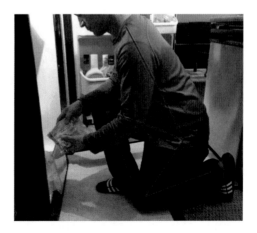

Reverse Lunge – Do this to also lower yourself to add variation for leg conditioning. The lunge is the single most important exercise taught in the program.

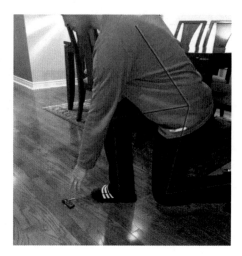

Reverse Stair Step – It helps to occasionally go upstairs this way because you are protecting your back by conditioning your hips and gluteus muscles.

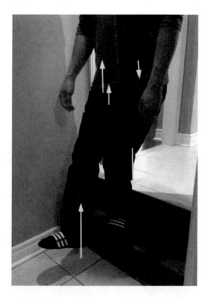

Standing Knee to Chest – Once you are able to develop enough hip and leg strength and flexibility, you will be able to use this exercise more often for dressing in your clothes.

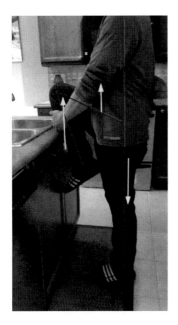 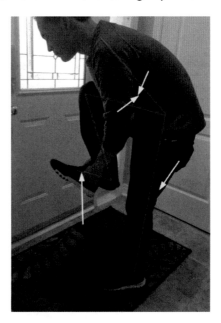

Forward Step with Hip Shift – A very effective way to go upstairs while creating hip flexibility and gluteus strength.

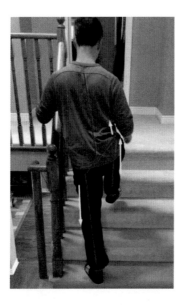

Foot Raise – This is ideal for putting on socks and shoes while strengthening your hip flexors and releasing your lower back.

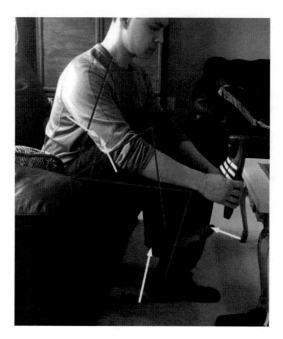

2018© SN Health Resources. Sherwin A. Nicholson.

While In Bed (either upon waking or going to sleep)

Most of us become very stiff in bed. This is when your back pain can really affect your quality of sleep. These are the exercises you can do to help relieve your stiffness, prevent tightening overnight and to help reverse the daily strain your back experiences.

Deep Squat Rest – Use this squat before you get into bed and as soon as you get out of bed.

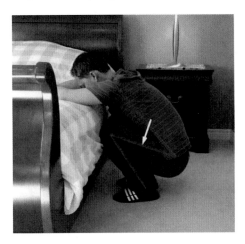

Kneeling Bow Rest – While in bed, this rest will help to release your back tension.

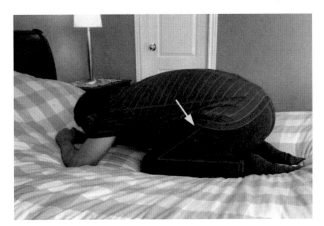

Seated Twist – This twist will help your lower and upper back *while you sleep*. You'll wake up with less stiffness.

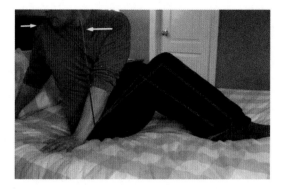

Pushes – If you have a pyjama pant with a secure waist tie, you can help relieve the tension on your discs this way. Remember to keep a pillow under your knees when your push.

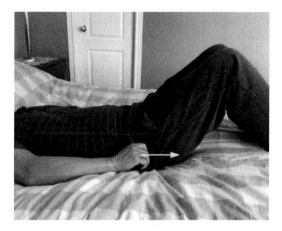

This exercise requires time and patience as you gradually begin to relax your back.

Lying Twist – You can release a very tight back and hip this way. Your upper back will also release from built up tension.

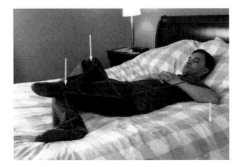 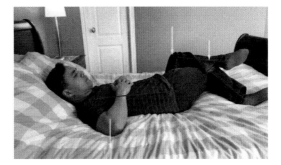

Abdominal Crunch – Do as many of these as you can to strengthen your core. This crunch helps to reduce any excessive anterior pelvic tilt that can cause pain overnight.

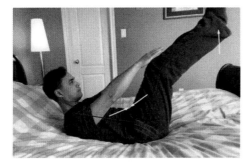

Seated Leg Cross with Forward Lean – Helps to open your hips, release back tension and excessive anterior pelvic tilt.

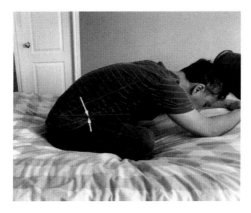

Deep Abdominal Crunch – More intensive than the abdominal crunch, it helps you to keep your core strong so your lumbar curve remains neutral.

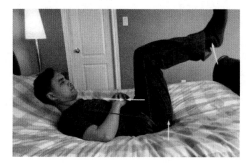

Standing Hip Shift (but modified in lying position) – While lying on your side, you can bring added relief to your hips and lower back as you hip shift. It's a great morning stretch to get your day started.

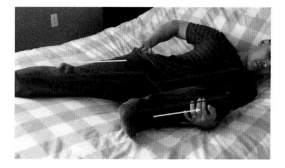

While Away

When away from your home, office or bed, here are some exercises you should do to help protect your back.

If you need to stand for extended periods of time, the following will counteract the tightness and weaknesses that may develop and hurt your back.

Deep Squat Rest - To relieve a sore lower back caused by increased pelvic tilt.

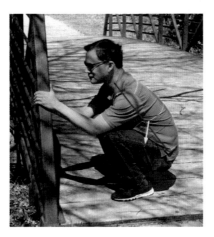

Standing Abdominal – To loosen up your back and create a more stable core. Even when you find that you have almost no time to do any of the exercises, you can still do this one.

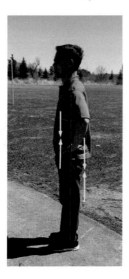

Seated Twist – This will protect you from back spasms and anytime you need to reach in awkward positions.

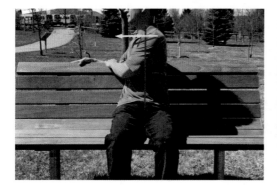 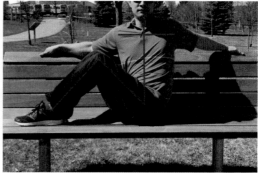

Leg Stretches – These are a must because your leg muscles generally tend to shorten as you stay active. The more that you stretch your legs, the better it is for maintaining your neutral pelvic tilt.

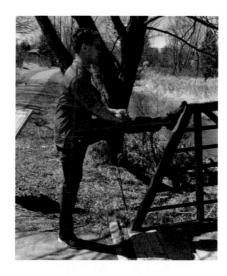

Calf Stretch – With constant standing and walking, your calves will become very tight and short. This affects your gait and causes back pain. Stretch your calf muscles often for injury prevention.

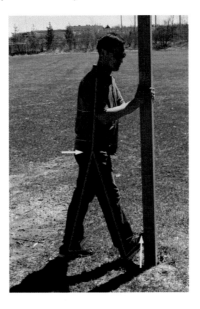

Quadriceps Stretch – This will release any excessive anterior pelvic tilt which hurts your back, facet joints and discs.

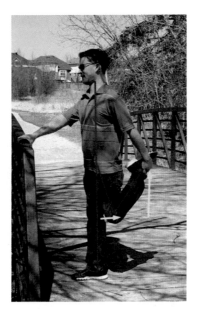

Rail Squat – If you can hold on to any stable support while away, you should spend a minute or two rail squatting. This way you can keep your glutes active and provide needed circulation to the lower body.

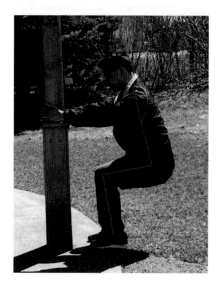

Hip Opener – This is an advanced exercise but it makes a big difference when you're on the go. Just doing a few will help your hips, hamstrings and legs which will protect your back.

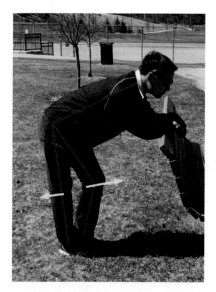

While Driving

Driving causes your lower back to lose its natural and neutral curve. It also encourages your hips to remain in a virtually locked position which is terrible for both your pelvis and lumbar spine.

Most of the time, your back is in a slouched position with a posterior pelvic tilt. This causes lumbar disc bulge which can be created from a poorly adjusted seat belt or a seat with little support.

Here are some ways to help counteract the imbalances and discomfort that driving can cause.

NOTE: Your priority is to always drive safely with your full attention on the road. *The exercises recommended are for the driver whenever the vehicle is in a stopped or parked position with the feet off of the gas pedal.* **Do not use these exercises while your vehicle is in motion.** Passengers can perform these exercises at any time to help relieve their back discomfort and also for pain prevention.

Seated Leg Rotation – Although you may not be able to fully rotate, the amount that you can rotate will help to keep your hips from becoming stiff and will also boost leg circulation.

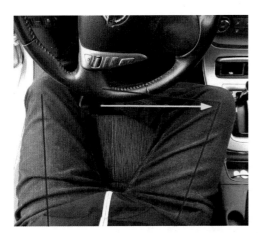 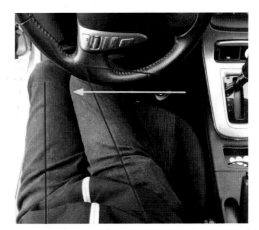

Seated Twist – Twisting will help you to keep your spine straight and active to minimize relaxation and slouching.

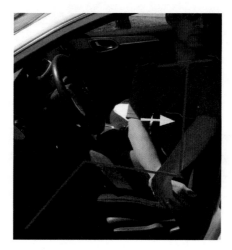

Seated Knee Raise – This will help keep your hip flexors active and improve leg circulation. It also helps to arch your lumbar spine when it is common for your lower back to slouch backwards.

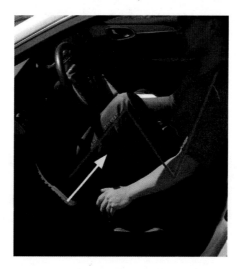

Seated Hip Shift – It helps to practice these shifts often when increased driving distances cause your hip and back muscles to shut down. Contracting these muscles will relieve a lot of discomfort for you and will allow you to drive more comfortably during those long trips.

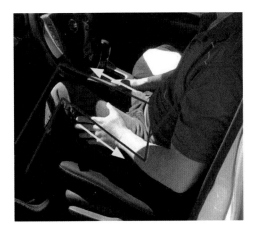 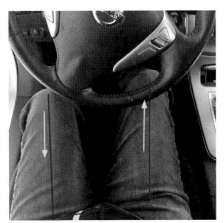

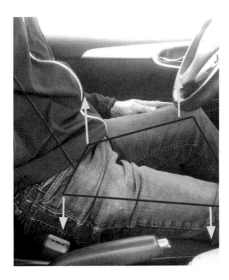

2018© SN Health Resources. Sherwin A. Nicholson.

Seated Leg to Chest – Relieve your risk of Sciatica and Piriformis pain while allowing better blood flow to your legs.

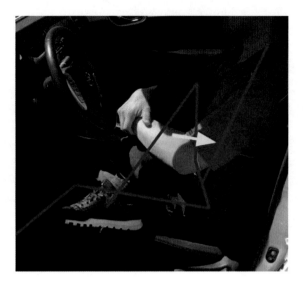

Standing, Walking or Jogging

Having to remain upright for extended periods of time causes both your upper and lower body to fatigue.

This can affect your pelvic tilt which may strain your back and discs. In addition, while the muscles of your body are constantly in a state of actively contracting to help you remain upright; your leg muscles are very prone to become fatigued and tight. Imbalances and discomfort will gradually set in unless you use these exercises often.

The following exercises will not only help relieve pain, but will *allow you stand, walk or jog for longer times/distances in a more comfortable state.*

Deep Squat Rest – You should squat to help counter the anterior pelvic tilt that can be naturally encouraged during these active upright positions. Only a few seconds of deep squatting can help you to relieve your discomfort to allow you to stay upright for longer periods of time.

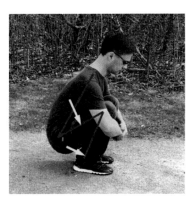

Leg Stretches – By stretching your leg muscles, you'll prevent them from tightening up and straining your lower back.

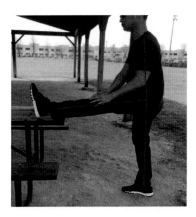

Calf stretches – Calf muscles are always tightening up in these situations. Be sure to stretch them often. You can't overstretch them if you stand, walk and jog often.

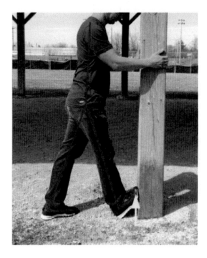

Quadriceps Stretch – This is key to preventing excessive anterior pelvic tilt which is a common cause of back pain while standing upright. It is one of the most important stretches to use at this time.

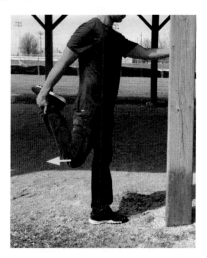

Leaning Hip Shift – You can keep your hips from getting tight while gently stretching your hamstrings at the same time with this very convenient movement.

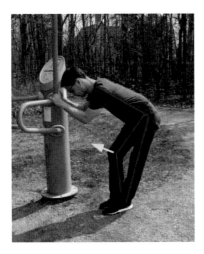 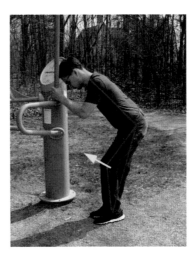

Hip Opener – This will help you to keep your hip joint stronger and more stable. This provides more support for your lower back and will help to release tension.

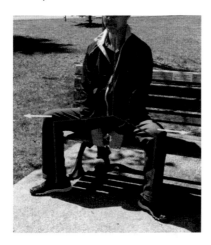

Double Leg Rotation (standing version) – It is important to rotate your femur often. This helps to release a tight pelvis and maintain your neutral pelvic tilt.

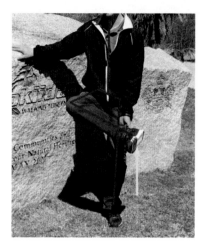 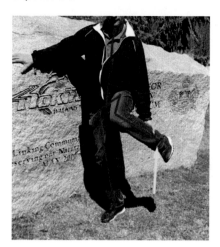

Standing Abdominal – Do these as often as possible. It only takes a few moments and very little time. It will help you to strengthen your core and relieve your back. Contract both your abdominals and muscles of your bum.

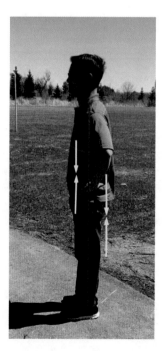

Holds (squat & rail) – You should be bending your knees often to prevent your hip and pelvis from becoming stiff. Holds are what will stimulate and activate your leg muscles more than merely standing or walking.

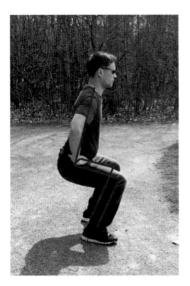 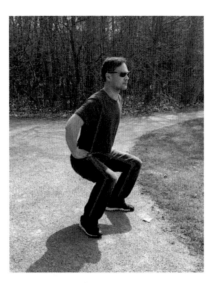

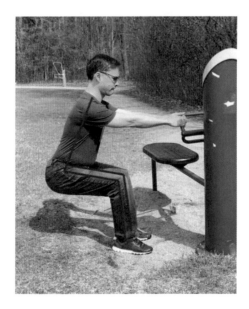

Lunges – If you are going to be upright for a long period of time, there is a good chance you'll need to either: lower yourself, kneel or sit periodically. This is where you should be taking advantage of the lunge to do this. You'll wake up your legs while keeping your back upright and safe.

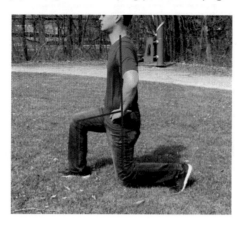

Standing Knee to Chest – If you find your back getting sore and don't feel you have the time to sit or lie down, do this as a quick way to stretch your leg muscles and to release tension in your lower back.

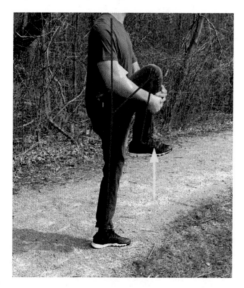

Standing Hip Shift – This shift will keep your hip muscles free and less stiff. It only takes a moment to do and can help you significantly.

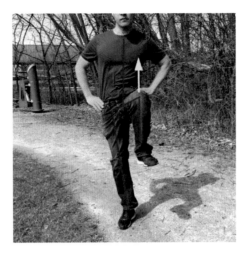

12 Modified Exercises to Help You with the Program

It is always preferred to perform the exercises *as originally demonstrated* but sometimes a modified version is required.

In situations where there is knee pain or difficulty maintaining your balance or posture, you can also use these methods to help make the exercise easier.

The modified exercises may be a better alternative to the original for some but where indicated; you may need to add an additional exercise to compensate for the differences.

Deep Squat Rest

If you have any difficulty with this exercise, here are some alternative ways to achieve the same benefits of the exercise.

Using a Support for Balance

If you find it difficult to keep your balance, use any support to help hold yourself up initially. Ideally it is better to squat unassisted but you can use a support to help get you started. **Your feet do not have to stay flat on the floor.**

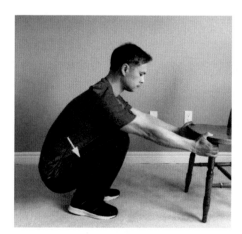

Heel Support for Balance – If you have very tight calf muscles (*which worsen back pain*), it's helpful to place a strip of wood or some books under your heels to help you stay balanced. In this case, you should spend *additional* time stretching your calves. Tight calves can compromise your posture and gait which also strain your back.

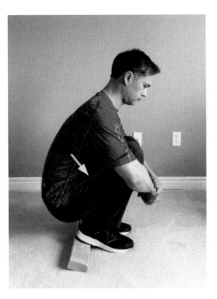

Using a Wall for Balance – Lean against a wall as a safer way to squat to avoid falling backward. You can also use it as a way to rest against to help you extend your time squatting.

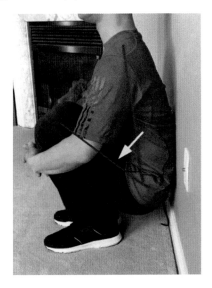

Lying On Your Back (to minimize knee pain) – By lying on your back, you can protect your knee joint. You'll need to stretch your calves in addition to have the same benefits of the Deep Squat.

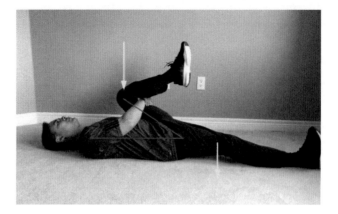

Seated Lunge

If you would like a gentler way to lunge while sitting, you can just lower your knee down to the side while *optionally extending your thigh behind your hip line*. This may be more comfortable or convenient for you. By doing this, you may be able to hold this pose for a longer time. Once you become accustomed to this lunge, be sure to progress to the full Seated Lunge extension as intended.

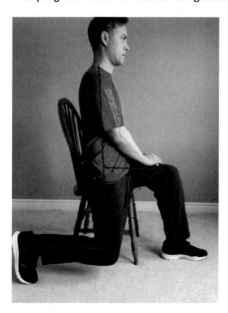

Seated Twist

In this exercise, it is better to rely on the muscles of your upper and lower back to help you rotate your body to the side. Holding unassisted to each side will help you develop the rotational strength necessary for reducing your pain (especially from back spasms).

Using your arms for assistance – If you need to, you can use your arms to help you twist. It is not necessary to use much force to twist. Just rotate enough with your arms *so that you can still feel the muscles of your back facilitating the twist* rather than your arms.

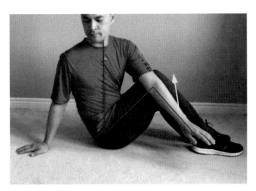

Lying on your side (for back support) - Lying sideways essentially allows even more of the twist to occur. *Once you can feel your upper body rotate easily, you should return to the original exercise instead of the modified method.*

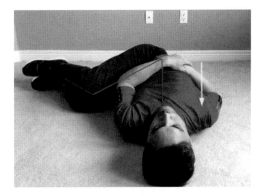

Calf Stretch

There are numerous ways to stretch your calf muscles these days. You are free to stretch them however you prefer. The non-modified method is preferred simply because a support is used to keep balance and both feet are stretched at the same time to prevent injury.

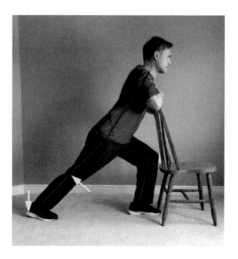

Lying Twist

Use the assistance of a cushion or a wall to help you to gradually twist. You can control the amount of the stretch and help to increase the amount of time you prefer to spend twisting.

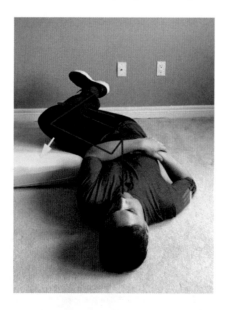

Hangs

If you have the strength, you can hang using your hands or your elbows if it's easier. *Just be sure not to fall and to keep your knees bent and in front of you.*

What I don't recommend is hanging upside down using inversion traction. The time required to feel the benefit of the relaxation is outweighed by the increased blood pressure delivered to your head.

If you have access to a corner or your kitchen counter you can do a partial hang this way. Depending of course on your upper body strength, this may or may not be practical.

If you lie down on a carpet floor or any surfaces that can help keep you immobile, you can ask someone to help you by gently pulling on your legs (knee bent) for a minute or two. This may be a better way for you to relieve some very tight muscles that are putting a lot of pressure on your spine.

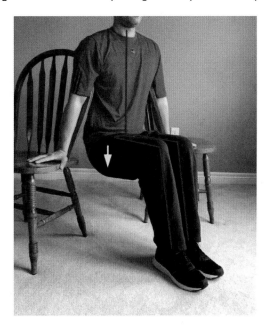

Abdominal Crunch or Deep Abdominal Crunch

Crunches are not very enjoyable to do. Here is a way to help you get going easier. You can simply lie on your back with your arms out to the sides for balance. Bend your knees and slowly lift them just a few inches from the ground. Then bring them to your chest and hold. You can use a rocking motion to help strengthen your abs also.

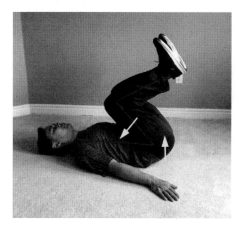 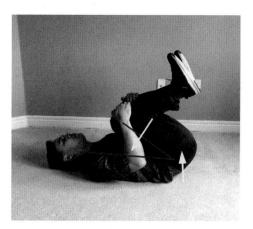

Seated Leg Cross with Forward Lean

If you have knee issues, you can simply rest your bent legs further out. *Only lean if you can.* If you do lean, try to *contract your abs* to lead you into it. Try to press your belly button *downwards* rather than your chest.

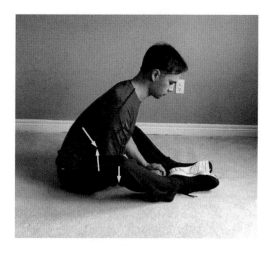

Plank with steps

Doing the Plank can be hard for some people, especially while stepping. You can begin by stepping while standing. Then you can progress by leaning on a support. Then just while on all fours with a simple lift.

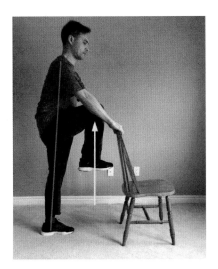 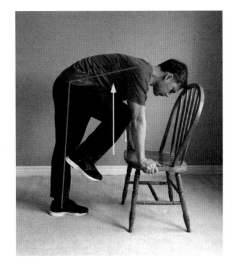

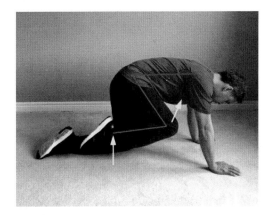

Outside Hip Stretch

This is a challenging stretch. If you would like an easier way and to have the same benefits, do it while sitting upright instead.

Begin with sitting upright but bring one bent leg inwards and in front of you instead. Hold and apply a slight forward lean. Try to contract your abs and hip flexors so as to focus on bringing your belly button *downwards* and **not by just leaning forward only**. *Do this for both legs.* ***Don't pull yourself forward.***

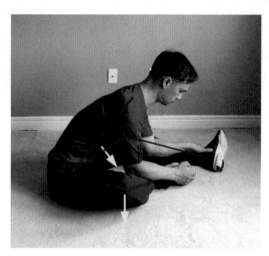

Abdominal Leg Press

If you find that using both legs at the same time is too hard, you can just use at a time without footwear.

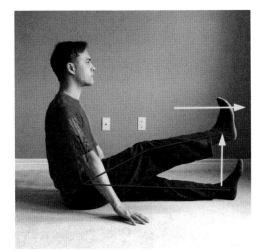 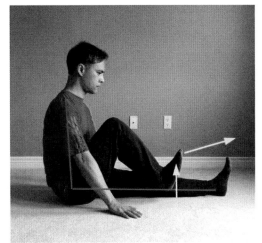

10 Custom Exercise Plans for Everyday Activities

Although it is recommend that you follow the order of the exercises, you can also use the following exercises *whenever you are active. They will help you stay active safer, longer and with less discomfort.*

For some exercises, you may find them challenging to do. Be sure to follow the Program in order *separately from the activity,* they will become easier for you.

Below I have listed **10** common activities in which there are **5** exercises for each one. They are taken from the Program for you to use *while active.* It will be beneficial for you to use them just prior, in the middle, and at the end of your desired activity. **This will be indicated below**.

Only the 5 most practical exercises are chosen so as to limit your time away from your actual activity. This is to maximize your own time while staying more conditioned and safe from back pain.

NOTE: Before you practice these specific exercises, be sure to continue with the Program. *Do not do these 5 only as an alternative to the Program.* **To achieve long term relief from back pain, the priority should be the full Program.** The **5** exercises listed for each activity are only intended to support your back during the activity and *will not be sufficient* for long term pain relief.

The times suggested below can be varied. Feel free to adjust them for greater convenience provided that they are not minimized or omitted.

b/d/a – <u>b</u>efore/ <u>d</u>uring/ <u>a</u>fter the activity.

Standing, Walking or Jogging

1. Quadriceps Stretch – b/a – 30 seconds per leg

2. Calf Stretch – b/d/a – 15 seconds per leg

3. Leaning Hip Shift – b/a – 1 minute

4. Standing Abdominal – b/d/a – 10-15 seconds

5. Standing Hip Shift – b/a – 10-15 seconds

If you prefer not stop in the middle of your walk or jog, you should then increase the before and after times to compensate. However, stopping will allow you to remain engaged in your activity longer.

If your activity however lasts for more than 15 minutes and you chronically experience back pain, then it is advisable to take the time to stop in between.

Weight Training

1. Deep Squat Rest –b/a – 1 minute

2. Seated Twist – b/a – 30 seconds per side

3. Leg Stretches – b/a – 1-2 minutes per side

4. Hip Opener – b/d/a – 10-15 seconds

5. Active Leg Press – b/a – 1 minute

Be sure to add lunges to part of your regular weight training routine. With or without dumbbells are safer for your back than using a barbell.

Golf

1. Quad Stretch/ Calf Stretch –b/d/a – 1 minute per leg

2. Leaning Hip Shift – b/a – 30 seconds

3. Standing Abdominals – b/d/a – 10-15 seconds

4. Lunge w/ Reverse Kneel – d – anytime you must lean down

5. Standing Hip Shift – d/a – 15 seconds

6. Lying Twist (while standing) –b/d/a – 15 seconds per side

7. Deep Squat Rest – b/a – 1 minute

Because golf can be very stressful on your spine, it is better to perform at least 6 exercises.

Gardening/Landscaping

1. Lunges w/ Reverse Kneel – d – anytime you must lower yourself

2. Lying Twist –b/d/a – 15-30 seconds per side

3. Quadriceps Stretch – b/d/a – 30 seconds

4. Leaning Hip Shift –d – 15 seconds

5. Hip Opener – d – 15 seconds

It is very common to become very sore from gardening or landscaping. These exercises will help you to extend your time while you work.

Snow Shovelling

1. Deep Squat Rest –b/d/a – 30 seconds

2. Seated Twist (while standing) – b/a – 15-30 seconds per side

3. Leaning Hip Shift –b/d/a – 30 seconds

4. Squat (holds, circles, steps & walks) – d – while shovelling

5. Standing Hip Shift – b/d/a – 15 seconds per side

Shovelling or digging fatigues virtually every muscle in your body. *It is vital to rest often*. Alternate with light and heavy loads and with a smaller sized shovel instead.

It is better to *always lower yourself down to the load than to bring it up*. Keep the shaft of the shovel close to your hip for support and leverage. Keep your knee bent and back straight at all times.

Repetitive Lifting

1. Standing Knee to Chest –b/d/a – 30 seconds per side

2. Squat (holds) – d – anytime you need to lift

3. Seated Twist (while standing) – b/d/a – 15 seconds per side

4. Seated Calf Stretch –d/a – 30 seconds per leg

5. Lunge w/ Reverse Kneel –d – anytime you must lower yourself

Lighter loads are always better for your back. Favour holding the object close to your waist. Keep your back straight and avoid any leaning.

Yoga

1. Deep Abdominal Crunch –b/a – 1 minute

2. Lunges – b/d/a – 2 minutes per side

3. Hip Shifts – b/d/a – 1 minute

4. Seated Calf Stretch – b/a – 30 seconds per side

5. Standing Knee to Chest –b/d/a – 30 seconds per side

By adding these muscle strengthening exercises, you can improve your balance and core. Because yoga sessions can be lengthy, it is beneficial to add these exercises to supplement your routine.

House Chores

1. Squat (holds, leans, circles, steps, walks) – d – during chores

2. Hip Opener – d – 30 minutes

3. Lunge w/ Reverse Kneel – d- whenever lowering your body

4. Lunge – d –whenever lowering your body

5. Standing Abdominals – b/d/a – 30 seconds

With enough practice, you will find it easy to use these exercises with your chores. The benefits of these exercises will come as the movements become second nature.

Driving

1. Seated Hip Shift – d – 5 seconds

2. Seated Twists – d – 5 seconds

3. Seated Knee Raise – d – 5 seconds

4. Seated Leg to Chest – d – 5 seconds

5. Quadriceps Stretch – b/a – 30-60 seconds

NOTE: As before, only do these while parked or stopped.

Dynamic Sports (hockey, tennis, soccer, etc.)

1. Deep Abdominal Crunch –b/d/a – 30 seconds

2. Lunges – b/d/a – 1 minutes per side

3. Advanced Hamstring Stretch – d – 30 seconds

4. Squat (holds, leans, steps, circles, walks) – d – while active

5. Standing Hip Shift (leaning and bent knee) – d – 15 seconds

Each sport will affect different dominant muscle groups. *However, your gluteus, core and hip flexors are the primary areas to keep conditioned to avoid back pain.*

If you add these exercises to your activity, you will help to prevent stiffness and tightening that comes with the sport you are engaged in. This will help you to remain *active for longer periods of time, avoid injury and have a faster recovery.*

How to Minimize Any Strain While on the Program

The Program will gradually move you out of your present discomfort, to challenging you to remain protective to avoid pain. In most cases, *you are already experiencing discomfort*. To help you minimize your pain while learning new exercises, you can use the following tips for support.

1) **Try to be careful with any current activities** that may be triggering or adding to your injury and pain. Although I strongly advise that you **continue** your desired activity or sport, it may be more helpful for you to either *put that activity on hold temporarily*, or to stop until your pain has become much more manageable.

    This allows you to recover faster, reduce your risk of injury and get a more accurate understanding of what may be contributing to your back pain. The rule of thumb for whether to use the program at the same time is that: *if the physical activity requires you to be very active when the curve of your spine is out of neutral position*, **then it is better to put your activity on hold**. E.g. *Too much bending, leaning, arching or weight bearing.*

2) **Warm up for a few minutes** prior to the exercises.
    Although not a requirement, you will find it easier to stretch and strengthen your muscle groups after a brisk walk, jog or warm shower. This will help as most of these exercises will be relatively new for you and will encourage you to use weaker and less balanced muscles that are not often used.

3) **Only perform the exercises partially.**
    You should not force your body to reach the final position of the exercise as seen in the final image. This will take time. Your flexibility cannot be forced. You only need to partially execute the movement each time. As your flexibility improves, change your position to that closer in the final image.

4) **Only do 3 different exercises at a given time.** If you need to do less, that is OK. When you are ready to challenge yourself more, only introduce a new exercise slowly and partially as before. *Slow and steady is ideal.*

5) **Use cushions, pillows, a soft carpet, soft and loose clothing, your bed** etc. to protect your back and knees. Gradual movements with a soft padded material may be necessary if you are in pain.

6) **Be careful with your pain medication**. Too much will numb your pain, causing you to exercise longer and more intensely. This can cause you to experience more discomfort and repetitive strain.

7) **Minimize any activities** that encourage you to do too much of the following: twisting, leaning, heavy lifting, sitting, slouching. Most of the time that you have to do these movements may be under less controlled circumstances as instructed in the program. This can cause wear and fatigue. Your body will take *a much longer* amount of time to recover and improve during the program because of this added stress.

8) **Gradually start each exercise in 5-10 second increments**. You can customize your own time but begin each exercise 5- 10 seconds in length at a time. For example, perform your first new exercise for only 10 seconds. Depending on the exercise, this short period is simply to help you establish, your position and balance and will begin to warm up your muscles.

9) **Repeat the same exercise** with an added 10 seconds in length the when you're comfortable. Each increase will help to condition your body to learn the new position, become more comfortable with the stretch, and to activate your muscles.

10) **Rest often.** Don't try to exercise *every* day. You should spend at least one day per week resting. Muscles and tendons need a rest period to heal and recover. Without this period of rest, you can risk a strain or sprain.

11) **Avoid repetitive injuries.** Must sure that when you do rest, that you don't return to any bad habits. Minimize or avoid excessive sitting, slouching or repetitive movements that can affect your quality of rest.

12) **Don't hesitate to skip any exercises** that you may find too difficult. If some are tough on your knees or hips or that you simply are not ready for them, then it is fine to work on the next exercise.

13) **Skip some if you must. If** you can't do some of the exercises, that's OK. Because of the number of exercises available for you to learn, there are many 'overlapping' exercises. There should be more than enough of the others to help compensate. The program is meant to be as flexible as possible for you (*no pun intended!*). It is not necessary to follow it strictly.

14) **Take advantage of your local swimming pool** when using the program. There are many exercises that you can do while upright in the shallow end of the pool. The added buoyancy will help to keep your upright, balanced and can lighten your bodyweight to reduce the strain.

15) **Be sure to spread out your routine.** Break up the exercises to morning, afternoon, evening. Do them every day with the occasional day off. This way you can avoid the weekend warrior mentality which can cause injury. The added benefit is that you will find the program less intrusive in your day/week.

16) **Always look for any opportunity to replace a typical movement** that you do each day (bending over), with an exercise (Lunge with/without Reverse Kneel). Make the program part of your life *instead of only something to add to your life.*

8 Common Back Problems You Can Correct

Tips and Support for Protecting Your Back

Here are 8 areas where you can learn how to help treat your pain. Each area comes with a list of individual tips and suggestion to follow. They are from my site Https://lowbackpainprogram.com and have been included below.

By following these suggestions, you will be able to add many different suggestions to the program to get yourself on the proper track for long term relief.

The Most Common Problem Areas Are:

1. Pain When You're *Sleeping*

2. Back Pain in the *Morning*

3. Managing Back Spasms

4. A *Safer* Technique to Protect Your Back

5. 7 *Habits To Quit* That Can Hurt Your Back

6. Back Pain from Sciatica and What You Can Do

7. 8 Mistakes to Correct to Relieve Pain *in the Morning*

8. Back Pain from Piriformis Syndrome

Pain When You're Sleeping

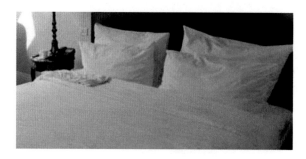

1. Use a moderately soft to a moderately firm bed

Most likely your bed should be adequate but there comes a time where some parts of the bed can fail. Check the bed tonight to see if there are any spots that sag. *Especially where your waist and bum rests.*

The bed will appear flat before you lie on it but after lying on it for a while, some parts over compress and give. You'll wake up in this sag, even sorer than when you got in.

Specialists usually recommend a firm mattress. However, this is to for **prevention** for those who are flexible, relaxed and have few symptoms. If you already have pain, a *softer* bed may help to cushion and absorb the stiffness that your body currently has.

Although a firm mattress is ideal, changing to one may or may not be suitable at the time. If your discomfort is already affecting you, a mattress change may be required. If it is not convenient or affordable, there are other solutions listed below.

2. Sleep on your side not on your front

Fig. 7.1

Tight Hip Flexors

excessive lumbar curve

relaxed lumbar curve

It is NEVER a good idea for you to be on your front (stomach) unless your back is pain-free or if there is a medical condition that requires you to lie down in this way.

2018© SN Health Resources. Sherwin A. Nicholson.

It is also better **not** to be on your back for now if it is **already** very tight and if your lumbar curve is excessive. Doing so will cause even more irritation and pain.

Most people have this very problem.

Check it out for yourself! Go lie down on a flat surface as seen in figure 7.1 above. If you have an arch under your lumbar curve so severe that you can drive a truck under, you have found a BIG problem for why you can't sleep well!

What is ideal is to be able to feel the floor or carpet just under your curve immediately as you lie.

Lying on your back can either cause or exacerbate an anterior pelvic tilt, that worsens disc and facet joint pain.

As seen in figure 7.1, it causes your tightened iliopsoas muscle to pull on your lumbar discs, thereby, creating the visible arch as seen.

When you are able to stretch out and relax these areas, only then will your lumbar curve be relaxed. Stretching your tight areas will help you lie down in any position.

3. Add lumbar support

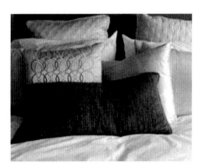

If you don't have an arch while lying down, lumbar support will help.

If you are the type that has more of a posterior pelvic tilt and shortened hip flexors (ex. slouching while seated), you may not have an arch when you lie down.

However, as you do lie down, your hip flexors will pull on your lumbar spine and create the same tension and discomfort as well. Use a small cushion to support a slight arch under your lumbar curve.

To help relieve the source of tension, use a small cushion to support a small arch under your lumbar curve.

If you have pain, the chances are you have an excessive lumbar arch when you stand. As you lie down, it becomes tighter as your back *tries* to relax (straighten out).

If you don't have an arch and it still hurts you, a cushion will ease any pull your iliopsoas may have on your pelvis that causes tightening. It also reduces any swelling from disc injury.

4. Add knee support

Always place a cushion/pillow between your knees. It keeps the knees apart and helps to relieve pressure off of the pelvis. Using a support underneath your knees is a great option. This help by relaxing your pelvis helps to reduce the same pull experienced in tip#3.

5. Keep your knees bent

If you must fall asleep on your back, use 1-2 pillows underneath your knees to help keep them in a bent position. Bending helps to tilt the pelvis towards posterior and reduce pressure due to anterior pelvic tilt. By maintaining bent knees, you also help to reduce the pelvic tilt experienced in tip#3. Again, this tip is for those who must be in this position instead of on their side.

6. Sleep on the couch or against a wall

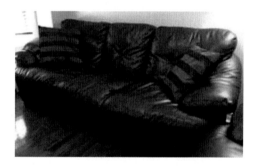

Use your trusted couch to lie sideways

If you find that you are rolling from your side, then onto your back, you will need to have a support. Use the upright support of the couch or a wall to remain on your side. It will keep you from rolling so you can stay asleep uninterrupted.

This approach, of course, is only temporary as your bed should be the primary choice.

7. Keep your room warm

Don't sleep with the room temperature down. It can make you feel too cold and reduce your circulation. Colder temperatures can make you stiffer and more uncomfortable at night. It also makes you prone to spasm due to your muscles tightening in response to the temperature change.

8. Dress comfortably

Don't under dress. You will feel colder and may have more frequent spasms or even tightness. Comfortable clothing will help you to feel warmer and will improve circulation to your back.

Don't forget to dress comfortably when you're spending anytime in the cold too. For example, after spending any amount of time out during the winter season.

You won't notice at first, but just a short amount of time in the cold will quickly make your joints stiff. You won't notice it because you're cold. By the time you're in bed, your muscles are already tense.

9. Practice relaxation *before* bedtime

Do's and Don'ts:

- Avoid strenuous workouts and activities that can tighten your back
- Minimize chronic couch sitting as they provide the least support
- Stretch more to help reverse any overnight tightness that develops
- Take a warm bath or shower to relax and boost circulation to all of your muscles

Follow these recommendations before bed. Your goal is to prepare your body for bed with relaxation and not from exhaustion. For some, their symptoms begin to feel better towards the night and worse in the morning. There are some very useful tips for morning pain. By relaxing before bed, your chances of a full and restful night are better.

10. And of course, exercise & stretching, but this way instead

The above 9 suggestions are merely part of the solution. This Program is here to help those with pain build a greater awareness of many of the strategies required to help overcome their struggle.

Retraining your muscles and joints to function more effectively is equally if not more. When you become properly retrained and reconditioned, you'll sleep much better.

Back pain due to mechanical issues such as disc or vertebrae injury can worsen your body's ability to regain balance. Muscle balance is what is necessary to prevent disc failure and joint injury. If it is not corrected properly, the imbalances will remain. This makes disc repair poor.

Back Pain in the Morning

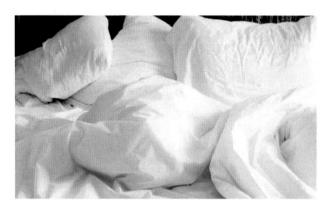

What can I do to stop from hurting every morning?

Below are the lists you'll need on how to begin so you can have a much better day with relief. Follow each one carefully. These tips will help to retrain you to move in a much better way that is safer.

Tips to Practice:

Upon Waking:

1. While still lying in bed, bring one knee slowly up to your chest and hug it with your arms. Hold for 10 seconds. Alternate with the other knee. The other leg should be kept straight as you hold your knee. Keep your spine straight. Do not forcibly pull your knee up to your chest. Keep alternating.
2. While still lying in bed, lie on your back. Bend both knees at a 90-degree angle. Cross your legs (one leg over the other). Hold this position and only allow both legs to slowly fall to the side. Hold for 30 seconds. Repeat in the other direction. Do not rush this as it will take time for any tightness to release.
3. While on your stomach, bend both knees upward and tuck your thighs under your stomach and chest. Hold for 1 minute.
4. Use gentle massage with your hands and knuckles around the muscular areas of your hips and lower back. Avoid direct pressure on the joint so as not to cause injury to any sensitive nerves.

After Getting Out of Bed:

1. Sit on the edge of your bed. Feet firmly on the floor. Bend one of your knees and bring one foot up on the bed. Your foot should be resting in front of you near your buttocks. Hold this position for 30 seconds. Repeat with the other foot.

2. Squat directly down on the ground until your stomach meets your thighs. Hold for 30 seconds. Get up slowly. Hold onto the bed for support and balance or squat down on a stack of books to avoid falling over.

3. Stand straight up and point both hands directly up to the ceiling while looking forward. Your hands, arms, spine and legs should be in a straight line. Hold for 20 seconds. Push up as if you are trying to reach the ceiling. Keep looking forward.

During the Day:

1. Allow 5 minutes of brief standing, walking or lying down for every 25 minutes that you are sitting.

2. When sitting, use a soft cushion and try to sit with as little lumbar support as possible. Your posture should be similar to someone playing the piano while actively sitting straight up and unsupported.

3. Avoid arching or slouching whenever sitting.

4. When picking up any heavy items or items that are low on the ground, bring yourself down to the object while keeping upright. Here you will be squatting into the position and not leaning over.

5. Avoid sitting and slouching for extended periods of time 1-2 hours *before bed*. (Ex. TV, desk work).

6. Wear only clothing that provides a loose fit around your hips. Denim jeans that do not stretch or tight pants can worsen your discomfort by limiting your flexibility.

7. Drink sufficient amounts of water to keep your discs well hydrated and to avoid muscle cramps.

Before Bed:

1. Incorporate as many of the exercises and stretches suggested above before lying down.

2. If recommended by your doctor, take an anti-inflammatory or muscle relaxant before bed. This practice should be minimized or done only if necessary.

3. Lie sideways on your bed with your knees bent and a cushion in between your knees. Avoid sleeping or lying on your back and never on your stomach. If you must lie this way, elevate your knees with extra pillows.

4. Maintain a warm bedroom temperature. Cooler temperatures can cause muscle stiffness and spasms.

5. Learn the Deep Squat Rest. It will test your stiffness. Mastering this movement will help to reduce your pain as it helps to increase your lumbar and hip flexibility. If you have difficulty with this exercise, you are at risk of poor muscle conditioning.

Managing Back Spasms

Note: If you are experiencing one right now or just want to manage them, be careful right now. *How you react affects your recovery.* Without proper help, the spasm will return in the *same way.*

For the best chances of recovery, follow in order so you'll have maximum benefit

- *Continue here for an in-depth discussion on <u>why your spasms return & what more you can do now.</u>*

1) STOP

Stop your activity and find immediate rest

This may already make sense, but many of us prefer to keep moving. **Some professionals actually recommend that you stay in motion,** *but if you are the unfortunate one to have a disc or nerve problem,* **then that is poor advice.** *You may end up visiting them for that instead.*

Don't try to actively work or move *until* you know the source of the injury.

A very common reaction is to keep moving but MAY be dangerous. Although this might *feel* helpful, it is important to determine whether your pain is more than just muscular in nature.

Why you should NOT move:

- <u>potential lumbar disc injury (rupture, bulge, degeneration)</u>
- <u>lumbar nerve impingement (pressure on the nerve)</u>
- <u>torn or sprained back muscles (overexertion, poor posture)</u>
- <u>facet joint wear or irritation (lowered disc height, over-extension)</u>

Moving when you have any of these injuries can cause further injury, intensifying the pain.

If you have a history of ANY of these injuries or suspect that your lifestyle may contribute to it (sports, work, inactivity), then rest is a better than simply muscling through it with medication.

Lastly with this first tip, you should know that you should also apply this caution to not just your back but also to your hips, knees and neck. Forcing yourself to move when these areas also hurt can be risky too!

2) LIE DOWN

Carefully move to a bed or comfortable flat surface to remain *temporarily* immobile

That spasm that you have is a nasty but very clear *warning sign* that you must *not* continue to move. Your body is literally 'locking up' to guard you against injuring **another** part of your back that is weakened or injured.

Although this 'locked up' muscle may hurt as it tightens, it is not usually the source of the injury.

By laying down, you can help to stop triggering these muscles and can reduce the intensity and duration of the pain.

You can lie on the floor using cushions and pillows as a support and just be patient. **It's better for you to focus on being somewhere calm so you can make yourself the priority.**

Remember though that this is only a temporary measure as prolonged immobility could make things worse.

Did your contraction happen while reaching for, or lifting something? Did it happen just out of the blue and during a very simple activity? If so, you should *follow this One Simple Rule to help reduce your chances of back spasms.*

3) RELAX & BREATHE

Consciously try to relax your muscles with slow, deep breaths

Seriously, I know this much easier said than done, but you NEED to do it.

If you learn to breathe the right way, it won't hurt so easily. Breathing poorly will move your rib cage too erratically and might trigger your back muscles again.

Try to relax your muscles when they are in spasm *with slow, deep and controlled breaths*. It's pretty painful to breathe deeply when you have a full attack, but it will get you to focus more.

We tend to breathe very quickly and shallow when we are in pain. **Shallow breaths or even holding your breath is a natural reaction, but will only add to the discomfort.**

Inhale slowly and deeply for a count of 5 seconds, pause 1 second, and exhale 3-4 seconds. Do not pause at the end of the exhale. Repeat.

Visualization will help by imagining a tight knot being unraveled as you inhale. Picture the muscles extending as you inhale to stretch your rib cage fully.

As the muscles are contracting intensely, they are also **over** contracting, making it counter-productive.

Since you have already stopped moving, you are now trying to *shut off* the muscles' need also to do this. Breathing deeply is key to relaxing a muscle which is *becoming progressively shorter and more painful.*

As you try to relax, avoid any movements that allow the muscle to shorten

Because of the intensity, duration and source of the injury, it is natural to react and to contract your body further. Even unwillingly.

To avoid this, focus on slowly inhaling while at the same time minimizing your movements. When in contraction, the reduced circulation and the build up of lactic acid makes you feel much worse.

- *Are you struggling with your Stretch Routine? Avoid these pitfalls to help control your spasm.*

4) Stretch

Lengthen the tightened muscle carefully and slowly

It's this tip/step that could reveal for you, how serious your back injury might be. If it doesn't take very long for you to stretch and relax your way out of the pain, then you most likely have a simple muscle associated problem.

Here is the bad news.

If you are finding this tip/step to be a hard to do and it is taking a really long time to do, you may have a much more serious problem beyond your muscular pain.

I don't mean to be the bad messenger but it's your body and you need to see this as an important moment to recognize what you underlying injury may be.

Try to lengthen your muscles by extending it, using movement opposite to the contraction of the muscle.

Lying on your side while crossing your arms as you hunch forward can help

Gradually increase the extension slight fractions of an inch and hold.

Extending take several minutes to accomplish. If possible, have someone assist you in with the extension. Maintain very slow, controlled inward and outward breaths to become calm and to relax, *even though you are uncomfortable.*

Note: *You are only trying to lengthen the muscle. Don't overstretch.*

Only allow very slight increments. By increasing the length of the muscle, you will relieve that muscle. You'll also reduce the injury to the area that the muscle is trying to protect.

Alternate periods of stretching with short rest pauses. Don't allow the muscle to contract during your rest phase as it may start again.

Reducing the intensity of the contraction can take anywhere from several minutes to hours if necessary. The degree of injury is a major factor. *Each time that you attempt to relax and lengthen the muscle, it will try to respond by tightening up.* Holding your position will help you avoid this.

If you have taken a very long time to use this tip for your pain, then please consider medical help initially. My site is loaded with lots of help for you also **but you should also get your doctor's support.**

5) Treatment

Treat the area 4 ways:

Tip #5 is to help to avoid triggering into another episode and tip #4 again.

Without treatment, the muscle that you just spent time relaxing, may re-tighten

i) Massage

You may, of course, need assistance with massaging since it will be hard to assist yourself.

Gentle massaging **along the length and sides of the muscle** will help by soothing the pain and allowing the muscle to relax slowly even more. **Your aim is to massage not just for comfort but to help improve blood flow** to the muscle itself.

Massage helps to increase oxygen circulation and will reduce the painful buildup of lactic acid.

Don't go nuts and massage your back like you are at the spa now. This massage is mainly for blood flow. If you over do it, you'll aggravate the problem and can also risk putting pressure on a disc or joint problem.

Avoid massaging if you suspect that your sore muscle is directly over the source of injury.

This would include an injured disc, joint, nerve or sprained muscle. You don't want to re-aggravate an injured joint or nerve with massage.

ii) Pain Medication

Be careful regarding the risks of relying on painkillers. It is a risk when it is your 'go to' so that's why it's not recommended until now and ONLY sometimes.

If the pain is severe and mobility is difficult, muscle relaxants, anti-inflammatory or anti-spasmodic medication may be required. **Use with caution and only if needed.**

There will be times when a muscle relaxant (such as baclofen or methocarbamol) may seem like the only effective method. Please use caution as these drugs along with other relaxants have their side effects.

Medication will only address the pain, not the source. By not treating the cause, your spasm is very likely to return.

Numbing effect

Pain medication also has a "numbing" effect (desensitization). The effect can mislead you to believe that your symptoms have been treated when in reality, you simply cannot feel them. Desensitization may allow you to prematurely return to the activity or lifestyle that may have caused your spasm.

I have heard a lot of people do this too often only to end up with both permanent soft tissue and bone injury. **If you numb these areas with drugs, they can't warn you anymore.**

When these nerves (muscular and lumbar) have become temporarily 'desensitized', you are more likely to re-injure yourself without your awareness.

Minimize our dosage

To help with your recovery, it is more effective to take a minimal dosage of pain medication such that you can still be *aware* of your discomfort. By doing this, you will have much better awareness and control of your recovery as your injury resolves. This will require a longer recovery time but will minimize your likelihood of premature injury and pain.

iii) Apply a Cold Pack

For the first 48-72 hours, carefully apply a cold pack to the area to reduce any inflammation present. *Protect the skin from any risk of ice burn with a thin towel before applying the pack.* Apply for 20 minutes and use every 1-2 hours as needed.

Caution: Not everyone benefits from a cold pack. If you find applying cold only numbs your pain while you are *still* stiff, then either reduce the length of time you apply it, or avoid cold treatment. Some people are more likely to feel even stiffer with cold treatment. The goal is to relax the muscle, not shock it.

I recommend that you go with what works for you. Personally, I prefer heat instead, but everyone has their own preferences.

iv) Apply Moist Heat

After 72 hours, carefully apply moist heat. A wet towel or warm shower will help. It is important to improve circulation to the injured muscle for it to recover and function well.

Caution: With heat, you want to avoid applying too much as this can increase swelling. If the heat causes an inflamed joint to swell, you will be re-injured.

6) REPLENISH

Rehydrate and rebuild your nutrient stores

Make sure that you are drinking enough fluids as dehydration and loss of electrolytes affect the length and success of your recovery. Low blood calcium, magnesium and potassium levels can affect some people who suffer from spasms.

These levels will fall drastically during intense exercise and can contribute to the problem of muscle contractions. If you allow these conditions to become chronic, you end up with muscle imbalances which will put your back at risk again.

Companion Guide
A very good friend of mine told me about her chronic nightmares of spasms and pain. She tried everything only to finally resolve them by increasing her calcium, magnesium and potassium levels adequately with a supplement. It didn't take long for her to feel a lot better. She said it was like night and day. It's definitely worth a try if you haven't considered it yet?

7) VISIT YOUR DOCTOR

See your doctor for these potential underlying illnesses

Don't just treat a back spasm as temporary discomfort. It may not merely be muscular in nature as they are often a big warning sign.

There may be something more serious that you are not aware of. This may be what your body could be reacting to.

In cases where treatment does not help, it is possible that you may have a disc issue such and a bulge or herniated disc. It is important to know <u>when you should see a doctor</u> *to diagnose any serious injury that may be an underlying cause.*

- Herniated Disc
- Spinal Stenosis
- Arthritis of the Spine
- Lordosis
- Scoliosis
- Spondylolysis
- Spondylolisthesis

8) PROTECT YOURSELF

Avoid re-injury and recondition your muscles

I hope that you have reached this final Tip. Most people actually do this step, but very poorly if at all.

For tips 1-7, you can more or less memorize them, recall them and practice them well. Please commit them to memory ASAP. Thank you.

However, if you forget about Tip #8, you'll be visiting Google, this page, the medicine cabinet or your doctor too many times and that will suck.

Treatment requires persistent and careful attention for <u>those who experience spasms repeatedly</u>. It is important to monitor your lifestyle activities to know what may bring them on.

After recovery, it is natural to assume that your spasm occurred as a result of a weak muscle or set of muscles groups.

Avoid rushing into the 2 most common mistakes for treatment

78
2018© SN Health Resources. Sherwin A. Nicholson.

MISTAKE #1. Do not to rush into basic strengthening exercises such as sit-ups, crunches or lower back extensions. *This may help for some, but* ***in most cases, these areas are already tight, short and strong.*** Tightness and overly strong muscle conditioning is usually the case with the lower back and hamstrings.

MISTAKE #2. Simply resting and returning to your daily whatever. *Weren't you doing this JUST BEFORE it happened? No my friend. There needs to be a plan and you are here for actual solutions right?*

Observe the <u>degree of your pelvic tilt</u>. The three common positions are neutral, anterior and posterior. An excessive angle (usually as a result of imbalances from a tight rectus femoris, psoas major or hamstring) can trigger another spasm.

Exercises such as sit-ups and crunches can help but should not be done first as they are considered as *isolation* type exercises. *They do not condition the core muscle groups to protect you. If you are in need of some specific exercises,* <u>begin with these 10 exercises.</u>

Muscles that are likely to contract during a back spasm include:

- Latissimus dorsi
- Internal abdominal obliques
- Psoas major
- Iliacus
- Quadratus lumborum
- Erector spinae

If you spend long hours of sitting in the office, driving, and at home on the couch, you can **easily** trigger another episode. This can be caused by<u> adaptive shortening syndrome</u>.

A Safer Technique to Protect Your Back

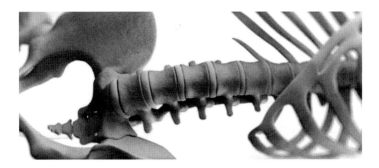

There is something we all do but shouldn't

We bend down the wrong way

Incorrect bending leads to disc injury

We rarely do it in a safe and balanced way. Not only is there unbalanced pressure on your back when you lean over, but also when rising up and it's harmful.

An unnatural curve in the lower back is also more likely to occur when you do this.

Take a look at the first image below. You can see a slight curve in my lower back when reaching downward. Observe in the picture where my elbows and hips are relative to one another (red arrows).

Most of us do not experience pain with this method because there is enough disc height and cushioning in between each vertebra. Lifting relatively light objects aren't usually risky.

However, if you find yourself constantly doing this, you're creating <u>unbalanced disc pressure, wear and degeneration</u>. Your hip muscles will no longer remain active, and a poor pelvic tilt will cause a disc bulge. Lifting anything at this time just makes it all worse.

The Wrong Way

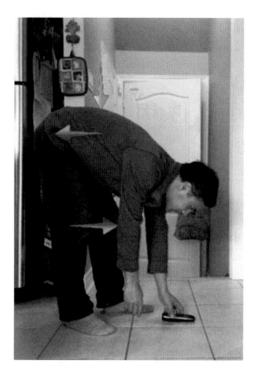

Over time, this becomes progressively risky for your spine.

The Right Way

There is a better way you can protect yourself easily. It retrains you and reconditions the muscles responsible for protecting your spine. With time, this will be a natural movement.

When you need to lean over, whether to reach for something or to pick it up, *follow this One Simple Rule:*

Keep Your Elbows Above Your Hips. That's it.

Now this time, take a look at my posture below. You can see that both my hip AND leg muscles are engaged. There is no bend encouraged in the spine.

The lower back muscles are recruited and activated along with the glute muscles. At NO time is it necessary for the level of my elbows to be below that of my hips.

The arrow at the top is pointing at the elbow, while the arrow at the bottom is pointing and the *hip bone.*

The weight of the upper body still remains above the pelvis which reduces the chance of a disc bulge that can herniate or trigger a spasm. Notice how the upper body has only leant over at a fraction of the angle of the first image. I can still maintain a neutral curve, which is key.

Keeping your leg muscles engaged in this movement prevents injury.

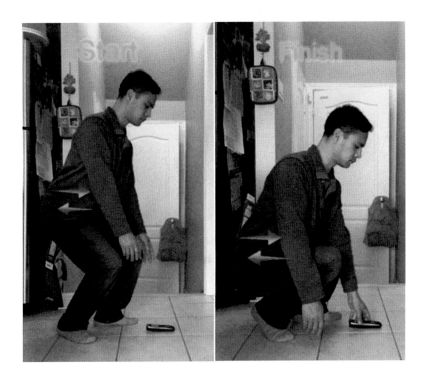

This is a much safer and preferred alternative to leaning over. If you keep yourself aware of this rule, then you force yourself to consciously bend at the hips, the knees and not the back.

Look at the benefits:

- Your leg and hip muscles are activated and moving.
- There is much less effort and strain on your body and spine
- You will reduce your chances of spasm and injury dramatically
- Lifting this way becomes very easy to do.

If you have difficulty performing this simple rule, you most likely have back issues. But you shouldn't avoid it.

Avoiding this method can make you more prone to both acute and chronic lower back pain. If you would like to pursue further help for this problem, this website provides <u>a wealth of information and support to treat your pain.</u>

To protect yourself from injury, keep aware of maintaining the following:

1. Minimal bending, twisting and arching of the spine
2. Keeping your pelvis neutral and stable
3. Engaging your leg muscles, specifically your gluteus muscles
4. Lowering your hips as you bend

Point 4 is often the least performed but is very important.

Most people will bend their back while lowering their upper body down to a lower level. Although doing this can seem very practical and may not hurt you, it is very risky.

Moving this way can easily cause you to develop back spasms. If done repeatedly, without balance, control and with excess weight, you'll risk chronically suffering.

7 Bad Habits That Can Hurt Your Back

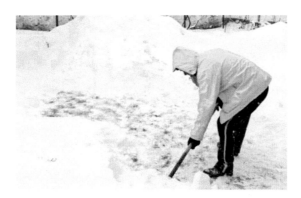

Our lifestyle is the biggest culprit for causing back pain

Your lifestyle has a major impact, next to injury or disease of the spine. The good news is that it is also one of the easiest areas to fix.

Let's look at 7 of the best areas to adjust with as little stress as possible.

When people think of lower back pain and lifestyle, they first tend to think that a sedentary life is the main cause. Although it can be a leading cause, others such as diet, stress, smoking, posture, proper lifting and amount or intensity of physical activity come in to play.

1. Avoid living a sedentary life

Sedentary lifestyles are never good. *Especially for your body.*

We are all guilty of falling into one at least on more than one occasion and sometimes, it's beyond our control. A sedentary life prevents and delays us from the proper conditioning that our bodies need to meet the demands of the day.

The strange thing about it is that at first it *feels* good to be sedentary, but with enough time you'll eventually feel much worse. Ideally, you *should* be feeling uncomfortable at first to be sedentary and much better after you avoid it, with activity.

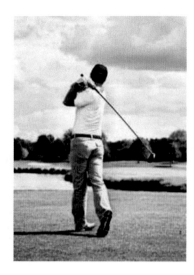

Teaching your core to become 'inactive'

The moment you go into a relaxed sedentary position of sitting or lying down, your core muscles effectively shut down.

Because the lumbar spine must bear heavy forces from our bodies, the muscles that support and protect it need daily 'activation' to function well.

Lack of basic exercise causes the low back to become stiff. Stiffness is usually worse in the morning while muscles can remain tight, weak, and sore for the remainder of the day. The discomfort and lack of mobility deter and discourage us from wanting to exercise these very same muscle groups that are affected.

It's a trap that is hard to escape

Sometimes you can fall into the trap of avoiding being active because you think you're better off resting. However, too much rest is also known to slow down our recovery efforts and even worsen it.

It is really from lack of exercise that leads to reduced flexibility, mobility and endurance. This is a tough cycle and habit to break.

Our spines are so forgiving of the abuse that we subject it to. If you only notice slight aches and soreness from time to time, rest or over the counter medications have most likely been your routine. Usually over the counter pills are adequate, and we continue with their use along with our current sedentary lives.

What we do not realize, is the amount of injury, long term damage and degeneration that can occur since we cannot observe direct damage to our spine.

By rearranging our priorities, investing much needed time to keep our backs healthy and stronger, and engaging in a spine healthy activity, we can reverse this cycle, accomplish more and enjoy more free time.

2. Creating a more active life

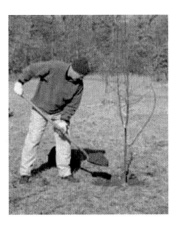

Active lifestyles are certainly what we all desire for our long term health and overall fitness and fulfillment. As with a sedentary life, there is also a strong correlation with an active lifestyle and back problems.

Many people believe that their active lifestyle is what helps to keep them pain-free. There are also many who are active yet suffer low back pain. It can be upsetting and discouraging as they are trying to stay active yet still suffer themselves.

They experience the same challenging cycle where they believe that with routine activity, they can keep their back from hurting while avoiding any sedentary choices. This leads to lower back fatigue and possible injury if they are following an insufficient approach to care.

When we think of an active lifestyle, we must not only think of a physically active one but one that places priority on the health and safety of your lumbar spine.

All activities, including sports and exercise, can be performed safely, provided that the body has adequately been conditioned to protect the spine first. Use caution with activities in which there is little emphasis on posture, strength, and flexibility of the spine and hips.

By focusing more on protecting your spine, you can gain more power, mobility and endurance that will result in better performance and enjoyment when you are active.

3. Lifting properly

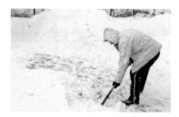

Proper lifting is essential as it requires a series of conscious steps and movements to move or carry something safely without hurting. Learning what is involved in proper lifting technique in step wise order protects the lower back and makes lifting a safer and more enjoyable task.

It takes time to develop but is very easy to learn. Over time, it becomes more effortless as the right muscles are activated and engaged naturally. Lifting technique is explained in the 'treatment and prevention' section.

4. Watching your posture

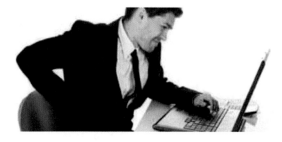

Posture is key to prevention of lower back problems. It is the first requirement before engaging in any task. It affects every area of your daily life and requires a conscious effort and commitment to maintain and develop.

It is vital that your posture is correct during activity as the lumbar spine must bear the most physical stress in virtually everything physical task done with the body. Poor posture is more common to have as correct posture can feel unnatural over time.

With discipline, it becomes easier and requires less effort over time.   Posture and a sedentary life go hand in hand and work together to contribute to making the pain progressively worse.

5. Quitting smoking

Yes, even smoking has an effect on your lower back. Smokers are three times more likely to develop it than non-smokers. The nicotine in cigarettes is known to cause thickening of the walls of our blood vessels such as our arteries. The effects extend to the blood vessels that circulate the flow of blood to the muscles groups that protect the vertebrae, nerves and to a lesser extent, the discs themselves.

Progressive narrowing of the blood vessels results in less circulation of protective blood cells, oxygen, nutrients and removal of waste products. Blood supply, healing and recovery are slower and less efficient. The potential for muscle injury and damage is higher for smokers.

6. Managing stress

Stress affects everyone regardless of pain, but stress does have a physical effect on the lower back itself. Numerous professionals, institutions, books, websites and other sources of information are available to assist us with the consequences of stress on our lives.

One way in which stress can affect our lower backs is on our ability to manage our time efficiently and also use it to exercise correctly. Sometimes with what little time that we have available. We tend to value exercise with the least priority and no longer consciously stay active, sleep, eat and maintain correct posture as well.

Another way is where stress affects our natural mental ability to relax. Here, the body becomes chronically tense and enters in preparation for a real or perceived stressful event. This generates significant muscle tightness in the lower back.

The lumbar area is very vulnerable to this condition become it is a very physically active part of our body. Muscle tightness in the lower back occurs as the body tries to stabilize the spine before the stressful event.

Stress also lowers our tolerance levels and raises our emotional response. We tend to find other ways to cope with the discomfort, either with more over the counter or prescription medication or by releasing our pent up and tense energy physically.

Existing physical stress, such as a previous injury or fatigue also exacerbates stress that is already present. We become too tired to exercise to treat ourselves. A chronic state of stress leads to chronic tightening of these muscles and minimal time and opportunity for them to relax and recover.

7. Keeping a strict but healthy diet

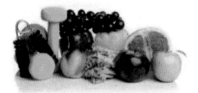

Diet is a very complex factor and sometimes requires professional help for it to become a valuable part of a back healthy treatment plan.

However, the most associated problem with back pain and diet is weight gain.

Extra weight places an unnecessary burden on the joints of the spine, hips, knees and feet. Extra weight stored in the midsection can cause the pelvis to tilt forward more thereby increasing anterior pelvic tilt. The tilt worsens as it causes the lumbar discs to bulge more and the support from the abdominals are limited and unconditioned. This weight causes lumbar imbalance, pinched nerves, sciatica, disc and facet joint pain.

Pain relief that is achieved with an exercise plan can be <u>more efficient and will progress faster</u> together with a successful diet plan.

It has been proven that by supplementing daily with magnesium, calcium and potassium, you can reduce chronic muscular pain. This applies to back muscle pain, spasms and tension.

Back Pain from Sciatica and What You Can Do

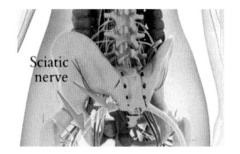

Sciatica is a very common type of radicular pain

Your Sciatic Nerve

It is literally a pain in your behind. And it hurts you when you least need it to. Both when you're either trying to work or rest. Heck, you can even feel it when you're standing.

Don't let it get to you. *There is help.* I have listed **12 tips** to help you feel better. But for now, it helps to know more about what it actually is and whether you really have it.

When your sciatic nerve gets irritated from pressure, you'll feel a very sharp, painful sensation. It can worry and scare you. It can make you feel like your whole lower body is in pain because of where it travels from your spine.

Since it's the longest nerve in the body, the intensity is pretty alarming.

It originates and exits from the bottom of the spinal column as a group of 5 to 6 smaller nerves. These nerves then combine to form the large nerve that travels down through the hip and down to the bottom of your leg. There is one nerve for each side of the body.

Pain from sciatica can be felt anywhere from the lower lumbar and sacral nerves, passing through the buttocks, down the thigh, leg and foot. It is also known as a <u>radicular form.</u>

People may be led to believe that this is a medical condition. It is not.

It is actually a way of describing the symptoms felt when pressure is applied in the lumbar region but felt on any part of this nerve from the lumbar column to the foot.

A Common Cause of Sciatica

One common cause is if you have a lumbar disc bulge. Too much pressure on your disc can cause the disc wall to weaken. As it weakens, part of the wall bulges out toward the nerve, causing nerve pain and numbness. It is usually the last two discs in the lumbar spine, the L4-L5 and the L5-S1. These discs compress the L4, L5 and S1 nerve roots.

We tend to abuse and wear out our lowest two discs. It even happens when you age, so it's important how well you treat your back in your youth.

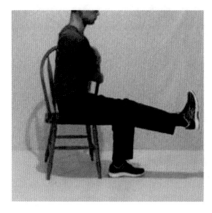

How do I know if I have true Sciatica?

Here is a quick and simple test you can down right now to help identify it:

1. Sit on a table or chair without leaning against the back rest
2. Begin with upright posture and your legs bent at right angles
3. Your thigh should be level with the seat and the shins vertical
4. Keeping your thigh on the seat, straighten the leg which has pain symptoms, elevating the foot

If it hurts and you feel like leaning backward to reduce the discomfort, then you have a possible pinched nerve. Extending the knee causes a pull on the sciatic nerve. If it is pinched, then the pull of the stretch will cause pain.

If your facet joint becomes irritated and swollen, this increase in size can cause similar nerve symptoms also. When there is degenerative disc disease, the disc and vertebrae can amplify the pressure. Degenerative conditions include osteophyte formation and osteoarthritic conditions. These changes also cause it to hurt even more.

Temporary Sciatica?

There are some situations where it is temporary, such as pregnancy and hormonal changes that increase swelling in the area of the nerve.

When yours is mild

Pain can range from slight discomfort to a sharp, persistent and debilitating sensation. The symptom depends on which part of the nerve is compressed. If the nerve is affected for a long time, the muscle that this nerve itself supplies may weaken and show deficiencies.

When it has worsened

If your condition is allowed to progress, the nerve can become damaged, and you may not be able to lift the forepart of the foot. Other problems of the foot include not being able to push off on the toes. An issue with walking may occur where there is 'foot drop'. This is where your foot may drop or drag on the ground as you walk.

What about Piriformis Syndrome?

It's almost like sciatica but not, and it comes from your behind and not the back. It's from a large muscle of the buttock, known as the Piriformis muscle that runs over this muscle.
Injury, swelling and tightness of your Piriformis can irritate this nerve, triggering a sciatic condition known as Piriformis Syndrome. There are some some excellent exercises available to alleviate this condition. Here is an easy and effective stretch that can help you.

Other Causes of Sciatica
- Disc rupture
- Osteoarthritis
- Osteophyte formation
- Pregnancy and hormones
- Poor lifting & Posture
- Excess weight
- Incorrect exercises and movements
- Poor back support
- Poor muscle conditioning
- Piriformis syndrome

Here are the 12 Practical and Effective Tips to Help You

1. If you have sharp pain, then stop and rest. Do not continue with your activity
2. Avoid Sitting for long periods and if you must, then move around every 30 minutes for at least 5 minutes
3. Avoid using a back support when you sit. If you must rely on them, then minimize your time
4. Rely on using only your posture to maintain sitting upright similar to a pianist
5. Don't sit on furniture with poor support: couches, sofas or anything that allows you to lean backwards
6. Lie down stretched out on your stomach or sides when your symptoms worsen
7. Use a cool pack against the lumbar area
8. Take an anti-inflammatory but only as a needed
9. Use a warm pack if the symptoms are not relieved with the cool pack
10. See your family doctor or health care professional
11. When symptoms are manageable perform simple stretches to relieve muscle tightness
12. Improve your flexibility and tightness in your buttocks areas to relieve nerve pressure

Back Pain from Piriformis Syndrome

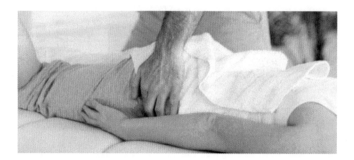

Does your pain feel deep in the sides of your buttock?

Does it get worse with sitting?

You may have Piriformis syndrome.

If it feels sore or tender when you put pressure on it, that's a sign also.

This syndrome feels <u>deep within the buttocks</u> and starts with the piriformis muscle. A lot of the time, it travels down the back of your thigh and then to the foot. <u>Sitting down for too long</u> will always aggravate this muscle, causing you to prefer to stand instead.

The piriformis is that large flat muscle along your buttock that is very prone to weakness and tightening, so taking care of it can seem like a constant battle. We cause it because of lack of exercise, stretching, compression from sitting, or even overuse which causes swelling.

When you allow it to become this condition, it gets *very* inflamed,<u> putting pressure on the large sciatic nerve</u> immediately beneath it. **Your irritated sciatic nerve is what is responsible for the discomfort you have.**

Solutions You Need:

Below, are some of best treatments for your pain. To prevent this muscle from becoming weak and irritable, **it needs routine lengthening and strengthening.** If your piriformis muscle is already healthy, it can quickly become a problem if you spend a lot of time sitting on it.

Before you begin:

1. Consult with your doctor to ensure an accurate diagnosis (vs. sciatica)
2. Avoid or minimize activities that worsen this condition
3. Use anti-inflammatories only when necessary
4. Follow glute stretches carefully and routinely
5. Hold your stretch for as long as comfortably possible
6. Practice as often as you can
7. Do not avoid stretching if it hurts in this region as soreness is part of the healing process

Follow these exercises to help you:

These exercises are very effective for gluteus/buttock pain.

Be aware that because you are trying to re-lengthen and mobilize a muscle that is already weak and tight, you will feel sore during and after the movement. This is normal, so do not be discouraged by any soreness as it will get better as the muscle lengthens.

A crucial part of the success of stretching is with the amount of time spent holding the stretch. Less than 30 seconds is simply not sufficient time for stretching any muscle. The muscle is only resisting your efforts at this time. Allow more than 30 to over 2 full minutes for the muscle to effectively relax and lengthen.

Try the Seated Leg to Chest Exercise

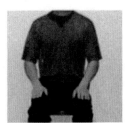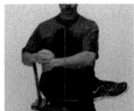

This exercise will easily lengthen the piriformis. It is easy to perform and can be done while you are at work or watching TV.

You will immediate feel a pull on the muscle. It will initially be very difficult to raise as high as in the image on the right. This may take days to weeks to achieve. Be patient as your degree of tightness relies on your commitment to holding your leg to your body.

Follow the full instructions on exactly how to perform this Seated Leg to Chest. They will help prevent you from using poor technique and will protect your lower back.

Seated Leg Cross

This exercise requires more intense effort to be effective.   It actively lengthens both sides at the same time.   Depending on which leg is on top, the intensity of the stretch will be experienced. This will initially require time to achieve the position indicated in the image on the right side.

To help, you can use pillows underneath the buttocks to help support you. Do not force this movement.

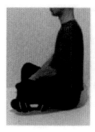 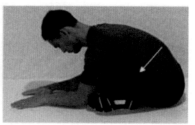

Take your time and ease into it slowly.

Follow the full instructions on exactly how to perform the Seated Leg Cross . The instructions will help prevent you from using poor technique and will give you lasting relief.

15 Tips You Can Follow for Chronic Lower Back Pain

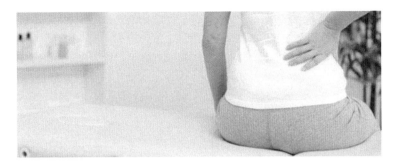

If managing your pain has become difficult, start with these 15 easy tips. *They will change your approach dramatically.*

1. Never Touch Your Toes as a Means to Test Your Flexibility

Never means never.

Never Do This

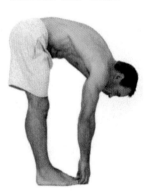

This is a terrible way to test for flexibility or for back issues. If *anyone* suggests this method, be wary of their advice.

Why? The action of leaning forward to touch your toes generates the most torque and force on the lumbar discs. **This is dangerous.**

By doing this <u>you will risk injury and spasms</u>. This movement does nothing to test for flexibility. The more that you bend or lean to stretch your hamstrings, the *higher* the <u>pressure inside your discs</u>.

You can <u>easily stretch these muscles without causing harm</u> to your discs. People who are not serious about <u>how to properly stretch their hamstrings</u>, will perform this action. They may be successful for some time but their discs will fail at some point.

At the other end of the spectrum, people who are fully able to stretch their hamstrings can perform this movement without risk of injury. This makes the test pointless to them as they do not need it in the first place.

If you were to design a way to deliberately <u>harm your L5-S1 disc</u> (the most important and vulnerable), it would include any method of leaning forward with your full upper body weight and holding. *I.e. touching your toes.* **Avoid this test at all costs.**

2. Engage Your Legs and Hips More than Your Upper Body

We *all* fail to use our lower body as much as our upper when required.

In fact, this is where the problem lies. If you use your leg muscles more to bend, pick up, reach or lower yourself, you will use your back less.

Before you consider leaning forward (which requires pressure on the lumbar spine), use your legs instead to bend to lower. This should be a conscious effort each time. It will not feel comfortable at first but it will benefit your health.

3. Do Not Rely on Your Lumbar Support when Sitting

Even the most ergonomic chairs provide minimal support. That is when compared with the support that your spine muscles, hips and posture should be providing instead.

A backrest is a rest and not a support. If you let your muscles relax while upright, then there is NO support contributed from the body. This means that your ergonomic chair is not helping your back. It only improves your comfort. You may feel better, but your chronic pain is still there.

The best way to sit is unassisted, upright, knees shoulder width apart, elbows close to the body, head up and with your eyes looking forward or slightly down. Maintain a slight arch in your spine with your chest slightly pushed out.

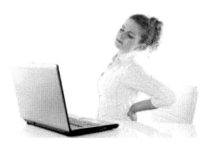

You can lower one thigh and knee down to the side for additional support. You can also use your arms to rest on your table or desk in front of you.

Use the backrest *as little as possible*. Only use it primarily to help tilt your pelvis forward toward neutral position. Sitting causes your pelvis to tilt backwards which can hurt you.

You will find this new position difficult to maintain and somewhat tiring. It does not mean that you should not continue it. It is a sign that your body is relying on rest instead of activity for support.

Over time, your back muscles will be able to sit upright unassisted with very little energy expended. You will feel much less sore when you sit and later when you stand. You will be able to sit anywhere and feel comfortable.

4. Exercise Your Supportive Muscles

If you do not exercise now or do not like to, then you will not be able to correct your chronic issues. No health care professional has even recommended an exercise free treatment exclusively.

The types of exercises that you should be performing are not the kind that you would imagine having to suffer through in the hope that they may help.

You are not trying to incorporate stressful, sport-like, cardio-class, extreme yoga workouts. That is not what you need. You need simple, safe and easy exercises that function to correct your daily movements and muscle imbalances.

5. Use Medications Wisely

It is between you and your health care professional how to use your medication. If you are using them as a supplement to pop whenever it deems suitable, then you are abusing both the drug and your body.

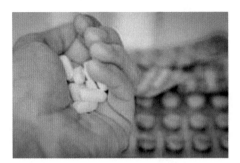

Taking medication to avoid pain may be necessary when you need it to function for important areas in your life. Taking them as to avoid other more effective treatments is not.

Don't dull your senses whenever it hurts. Use it as a sign that something more significant should be done. Sometimes we associate emotional pain with physical pain too often.

We find that by taking medication to avoid pain, we can help the emotional toll that comes with it. If you have been affected to the point of giving up on most treatments and relying on medication solely, seek help.

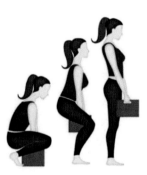

6. When you need to lift a heavy object, Hold it close to you, it won't mind

When lifting or carrying heavy or awkward objects, make sure to grasp and hold the object closely to your body.   It will help you to use your side as a support, thereby not relying only on your arms. It will also help to keep you balanced. Very heavy objects should not be carried if you currently have a disc problem.

7. Get down to it instead

Whenever you need to reach down to pick up something, do not bend or lean over. Bend at the knees and hips to lower yourself. Please follow this one simple rule from the How to Protect Your Back page for detailed instruction. It reduces your chances of a lumbar disc injury or back spasm. The exercise will primarily help to strengthen your leg muscles and improve your hip mobility.

8. Squatting, not leaning

When picking up heavy or large items, lower yourself as if you were squatting down on a chair and bring the object closer to your centre of gravity.

9. Your hips & legs are the problem, not the back

Keep your hips and legs conditioned by performing the Reverse Lunge. The reverse lunge is an exercise that you can do anytime you must lower your body. You can make use of this movement for example, when tying shoelaces, doing housework or anything that requires you to lower your centre of gravity.

10. Get off your... you know

Avoid sitting for extended periods of time. For every 30 min of sitting, spend one to two minutes standing. At work, use the opportunity to take bathroom breaks, get something else done, etc.
It helps to exercise the legs and to mobilize the hips.

11. When you can't... you know

If you must sit for long periods of time, then incorporate the Seated Lunge into your day. The seated lunge should often be done and especially if you are already experiencing symptoms of pain. This exercise helps to reduce your posterior pelvic tilt. It will also stretch the hip flexors. If you neglect these two areas, you will be prone to chronic pain.

12. Think before you move, even when you're not thinking

When you need to reach over or down to pick up or manipulate an item or object, position your body, so the object is positioned directly in front of you.

Avoid twisting to your side and never behind your (ex. reaching behind to the rear seat of your car to retrieve something.). This is a complex movement for your spine and will risk disc injury.

When you often move this way, spasms are likely. Unless your upper and lower body are well conditioned for this movement, you will more likely cause an injury due to the significant muscle imbalances which are there.

13. Better to know *than not to know*

Avoid the unnecessary use of over medicating to reduce symptoms of pain. Chronic use of acetaminophen and ibuprofen may alleviate immediate discomfort but will not address the root causes that lead to the discomfort.

By masking your discomfort with medication, you risk further injury by engaging in activities prematurely.

Minimizing your intake of pain medication will help to make you more aware of your present injury. Although this does not help with your discomfort, it will help to prevent you from further risk of re-injury.

Minimizing serves to extend your recovery time and increase your body's need to repair and heal. Excessive use of anti-inflammatory medication actually impairs the efficiency of your immune system. It is your immune system among other factors which are necessary for the repair process for your discs, joints, tendons, ligaments and muscles.

14. Clench away

Try to consciously contract your gluteus muscles (buttock clenching) before your rise from your seat or the floor. This action engages them in contracting before your quadriceps will.

This provides more stability for your pelvis and reduces lumbar discomfort. Healthy and responsive glute muscles are essential for relief. Chronic sitting 'shuts down' natural gluteus activity.

15. Stretch, your time wisely

Adopt a structured, progressive and safe method of stretching. Target muscle groups that have a known effects on the health a well being of your lumbar spine. Target your lower back, hips and legs. Follow this routine on a daily basis to ensure the protection of your joints and discs.

Be sure to commit the time and effort needed to follow these tips on a daily basis. They can all be done as part of your daily routine and require very little extra time in your schedule as you can perform them as part of your schedule.

For more detail on how to perform the exercises mentioned on this page, please see the section on one simple rule for pain, reverse lunging to help your glutes and doing the seated lunge when it hurts while sitting. These pages will help to ensure that you can perform these exercises correctly and safely.

Individualized Quick Start Exercise Charts

Tackle Everyday Activities or Concerns That Affect Your Back

When starting, you may find it a bit intimidating at first because of the number of exercises involved. Fortunately, the exercises are designed and planned to be very short in duration and by spreading them out throughout your day, they become fairly easy to follow and maintain.

It is better to begin in order from the first exercise to the final while progressing from level to level. This is the ideal way to recondition your hip, legs and lower back.

However, each of us suffers from back pain for different reasons. As part of the Companion Guide, there are **7 Quick Start Charts** to choose from to help get you started depending on your source of back pain. If your specific cause of your pain is not listed below, please follow the program in its entirety as it would be the most advisable method.

These charts are for helping you with:

- Your particular pain symptom
- The activity you experience pain the most often
- Getting you start as quickly and conveniently as possible
- Help you to progress out your discomfort quickly
- Keeping you focused

With the Quick start charts, each category has a specific order of exercises and the amount of time you may need to devote to each one. *Remember to use the modified versions when necessary.*

As with many others, you may find that your symptoms may overlap with more than one chart.

If you find that more than three (3) charts apply to you, it will be better worth your time to avoid the quick start charts and simply to follow the program in its entirety.

If 2-3 charts apply to you, then begin with chart that you feel you experience pain the least often.

Doing this allows you to take advantage of your current strengths and abilities. It helps to get you moving forward in your recovery when healthier muscle groups are already available.

When you find that you are able to progress through that particular chart comfortably and efficiently, move on to the next Quick Start Chart. **It is also OK to perform more than one chart at a time** but you may find it more time consuming and tiring for you. Any overlapping exercise between charts can be done once rather than in duplication.

Chart Rules

1. Follow your desired chart schedule outside of the specific activity. *You can use the 'ON THE GO' exercises as you perform the activity.*

2. Do a maximum of 3 exercises per day. You can introduce a new exercise when one *becomes too easy to do.*

3. Start at the top of the chart (easiest) and progress down to the bottom (most difficult).

4. Do **3** different exercises at a given time for *at least one week* or until they become *easy* to do.

5. Grey boxes indicate the Limited Mobility exercises, green boxes indicate the Progressive exercises and the blue boxes indicate the Challenging exercises.

6. The suggested frequency, duration and repetitions are only suggestions. Everyone varies in level of discomfort, injury and ability or time to recovery. *Please adjust to your own preference if necessary.*

7. Frequency refers to the number of days per week. Ex. 3 = Mon/Wed/Fri, 7 = Daily

8. Duration refers to the amount of time spent holding the final pose in the image. *If a time is not given, then holding is not necessary and you may work at your own pace.*

9. Repetitions refer to the number of times advised to repeat the entire exercise again.

10. Repetitions can either be done consecutively, or spread out through the day. Ex. Morning, afternoon and bedtime.

The Low Back Pain Program
QUICK START CHART
OFFICE WORK

Exercises (3-4 max./day)	Frequency	Duration	Repetitions
Seated Leg Opener	5	15 sec	8
Seated Leg Rotations	5	15 sec	8
Seated Twists	5	30 sec	5
Seated Lunge	7	1 min	5
Lying Twist	5	1 min	2
Abdominal Crunch	3	15 sec	5
Quadriceps Stretch	3	2 min	2
Seated Knee Raise	4	20 sec	4
Seated and Floor Hip Shift	3	15 sec	5
Seated Leg to Chest	3	30 sec	3
Leaning Hip Shift	4	5 sec	10
Hip Opener	5	-	8
Seated Calf Stretch	3	5 sec	5
Deep Abdominal Crunch	3	5 sec	6
Couch Splits	3	1 min	2
Reverse Lunge	7	-	10
Abdominal Leg Press	3	-	8

Duration: Time held in *your most comfortable* final position. Individual times are flexible and can be adjusted
Repetitions: Total number for each side. Ex. Left leg/side or right leg/side
Frequency: Total number of days per week Ex. 3 =MWF, 4=MWF+Sa or Su

The Low Back Pain Program
QUICK START CHART
STANDING, WALKING, JOGGING

Exercises (3-4 max./day)	Frequency	Duration	Repetition
Deep Squat Rest	4	1 min	3
Seated Lunge	5	30 sec	3
Leg Stretch	5	2 min	3
Calf Stretch	5	2 min	2
Abdominal Crunch	5	15 sec	5
Seated Leg Rotation (assisted w/ contraction)	5	15 sec	5
Floor Leg Bend and Shift	4	30 sec	5
Seated Hamstring Stretch	5	1 min	3
Hip Opener	5	1 min	2
Plank with Steps	3	1 min	2
Couch Splits	5	1 min	3
Standing Abdominals	7	30 sec	3
Squat (holds,leans, circles, steps, walks)	3	1 min	1
Standing Knee to Chest	3	15 sec	3
Standing Hip Shift	5	5 sec	5
Forward Stair Step with Hip Shift	5	5 sec	8
Abdominal Leg Press	3	15 sec	6

Duration: Time held in *your most comfortable* final position. Individual times are flexible and can be adjusted
Repetitions: Total number for each side. Ex. Left leg/side or right leg/side
Frequency: Total number of days per week Ex. 3 =MWF, 4=MWF+Sa or Su

The Low Back Pain Program
QUICK START CHART
SLEEPING

Exercises (3-4 max./day)	Frequency	Duration	Repetition
Deep Squat Rest	3	1 min	3
Seated Twist	5	30 sec	3
Seated Lunge	7	1 min	2
Hangs and Pushes	5	15 sec	3
Lying Twist	5	30 sec	3
Abdominal Crunch	5	15 sec	7
Quadriceps Stretch	7	1 min	3
Seated and Floor Hip Shift	5	15 sec	6
Seated Leg Cross w/ forward lean	5	30 sec	3
Seated Leg to Chest	5	30 sec	4
Hip Opener	5	30 sec	3
Couch Splits	5	1 min	2
Standing Abdominal	7	30 sec	3
Reverse Lunge	7	-	8
Reverse Stair Step	5	-	8
Standing Hip Shift	5	5 sec	5
Forward Stair Step with Hip Shift	5	5 sec	8

Duration: Time held in *your most comfortable* final position. Individual times are flexible and can be adjusted
Repetitions: Total number for each side. Ex. Left leg/side or right leg/side
Frequency: Total number of days per week Ex. 3 =MWF, 4=MWF+Sa or Su

The Low Back Pain Program
QUICK START CHART
AROUND THE HOME

Exercises (3-4 max./day)	Frequency	Duration	Repetition
Kneeling Bow Rest	5	1 min	2
Seated Leg Rotation	5	15 sec	6
Seated Twist	7	30 sec	2
Seated Lunge	7	30 sec	3
Quadriceps Stretch	5	1 min	3
Seated Hip and Floor Shift	3	15 sec	3
Seated Leg to Chest	5	30 sec	3
Leaning Hip Shift	5	30 sec	3
Rail Squat	7	15 sec	2
Stair Step	7	-	8
Hip Opener	5	30 sec	2
Seated Calf Stretch	3	10 sec	3
Couch Splits	3	1 min	2
Standing Abdominal	7	30 sec	3
Squats	3	30 sec	2
Lunge with Reverse Kneel	7	-	6
Forward Stair Step with Hip Shift	7	5 sec	7

Duration: Time held in *your most comfortable* final position. Individual times are flexible and can be adjusted
Repetitions: Total number for each side. Ex. Left leg/side or right leg/side
Frequency: Total number of days per week Ex. 3 =MWF, 4=MWF+Sa or Su

The Low Back Pain Program
QUICK START CHART
PHYSICAL ACTIVITY/SPORTS

Exercises (3-4 max./day)	Frequency	Duration	Repetition
Deep Squat Rest	7	1 min	2
Seated Lunge	7	30 sec	3
Lying Twist	7	30 sec	3
Quadriceps Stretch	5	2 min	3
Floor Leg Bend and Shift	5	30 sec	6
Seated Leg to Chest	5	30 sec	4
Hip Opener	7	30 sec	2
Seated Calf Stretch	5	15 sec	3
Plank with Steps	5	5 sec	8
Couch Splits	5	1 min	2
Outside Hip Stretch	5	1 min	2
Seated Leg Lift	5	5 sec	2
Advanced Hamstring Stretch	7	1 min	3
Reverse Lunge	7	-	8
Reverse Stair Step	5	-	12
Forward Step with Hip Shift	5	5 sec	8
Abdominal Leg Press	7	5 sec	5

Duration: Time held in *your most comfortable* final position. Individual times are flexible and can be adjusted
Repetitions: Total number for each side. Ex. Left leg/side or right leg/side
Frequency: Total number of days per week Ex. 3 =MWF, 4=MWF+Sa or Su

The Low Back Pain Program
QUICK START CHART
DRIVING

Exercises (3-4 max./day)	Frequency	Duration	Repetition
Seated Leg Opener	5	15 sec	3
Seated Leg Rotation	5	15 sec	5
Seated Twist	7	30 sec	3
Seated Lunge	7	30 sec	4
Abdominal Crunch	5	5 sec	5
Quadriceps Stretch	7	30 sec	3
Seated Knee Raise	7	15 sec	3
Seated and Floor Hip Shift	3	5 sec	3
Seated Leg Rotation (assisted w/ contraction)	5	5 sec	4
Seated Leg to Chest	5	30 sec	3
Hip Opener	5	-	10
Seated Calf Stretch	5	5 sec	5
Couch Splits	3	1 min	3
Outside Hip Stretch	3	1 min	2
Reverse Lunge	7	-	8
Reverse Stair Step	3	-	8
Forward Stair Step with Hip Shift	5	5 sec	8

Duration: Time held in *your most comfortable* final position. Individual times are flexible and can be adjusted
Repetitions: Total number for each side. Ex. Left leg/side or right leg/side
Frequency: Total number of days per week Ex. 3 =MWF, 4=MWF+Sa or Su

The Low Back Pain Program
QUICK START CHART
POST SPASM/INJURY/SURGERY

You must have your doctors consent prior to any exercises suggested here

Do not attempt or continue if you experience any sharp pain

Exercises (3-4 max./day)	Frequency	Duration	Repetition
Kneeling Bow Rest	5	30 sec	1
Seated Leg Opener	5	5 sec	5
Seated Leg Rotations	5	5 sec	5
Seated Lunge	7	10 sec	3
Leg Stretch	5	20 sec	3
Calf Stretch	5	30 sec	2
Lying Twist	3	15 sec	2
Quadriceps Stretch	5	30 sec	1
Seated Knee Raise	3	5 sec	3
Seated Leg Rotation (assisted w/ contraction)	3	5 sec	3
Rail Squat	5	-	5
Stair Step	5	-	5
Double Leg Rotation	3	5 sec	3
Standing Abdominal	5	10 sec	3
Lunge with Reverse Kneel	5	-	3

Duration: Time held in *your most comfortable* final position. Individual times are flexible and can be adjusted

Repetitions: Total number for each side. Ex. Left leg/side or right leg/side

Frequency: Total number of days per week Ex. 3 =MWF, 4=MWF+Sa or Su

Be Sure to Check Out:

- Frequently Asked Questions of The Program
  https://lowbackpainprogram.com/frequently-asked-questions/
- Commonly Asked Questions from Current Users
  https://lowbackpainprogram.com/ebook-support-faqs/
- eBook/PDF/Program Instructions on How to Use The Program
  https://lowbackpainprogram.com/ebook-instructions/

NOTES:

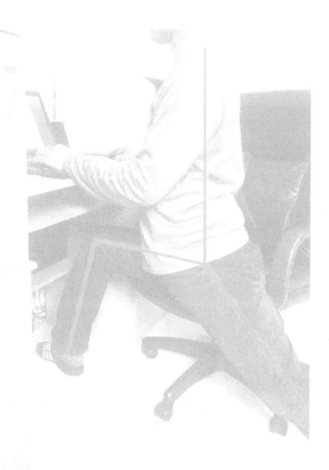

Made in the USA
Monee, IL
25 June 2021